Introduction to Program Evaluation

for

Comprehensive Tobacco Control Programs

November 2001

Goldie MacDonald, Ph.D.
Gabrielle Starr, M.A.
Michael Schooley, M.P.H.
Sue Lin Yee, M.P.H.
Karen Klimowski, M.P.H.
Katherine Turner, M.P.H.

DEPARTMENT OF HEALTH AND HUMAN SERVICES
Centers for Disease Control and Prevention
National Center for Chronic Disease Prevention and Health Promotion
Office on Smoking and Health

Suggested citation: MacDonald G, Starr G, Schooley M, Yee SL, Klimowski K, Turner K. Introduction to Program Evaluation for Comprehensive Tobacco Control Programs. Atlanta (GA): Centers for Disease Control and Prevention; 2001.

Acknowledgments

We thank the following people from the Office on Smoking and Health for their assistance in coordinating, reviewing, and producing this document: Karil Bialostosky, Linda Block, Monica Eischen, Lawrence Green, Corinne Husten, Mary Hill, Monica Manns, Terry Pechacek, Lisa Petersen, Scott Proescholdbell, Robert Robinson, Stephanie Staras, JoDe Walp, Eric Wiesen, and Leah Zinner.

The Office on Smoking and Health extends special thanks to Linda Crossett, R.D.H., National Center for Chronic Disease Prevention and Health Promotion, Division of Adolescent and School Health; Michelle Kegler, Dr.P.H., Emory University, Rollins School of Public Health; Bobby Milstein, M.P.H., National Center for Chronic Disease Prevention and Health Promotion, Division of Adult and Community Health; and members of the National Tobacco Control Program's State Evaluation and Outcomes Transition Team for their careful review of an earlier draft of the manual.

To better meet the needs of our state and local tobacco control partners, we evaluated this document for usability. We thank Jane R. Bratz, B.S.S., Bureau of Chronic Diseases and Injury Prevention, Division of Tobacco Prevention, Pennsylvania Department of Health; Susan Cummings, B.S.N., C.P.H.Q., Health Systems Bureau, Department of Public Health and Human Services, State of Montana; Cheryl Jappert, B.S., Division of Health Promotion and Education, Nebraska Department of Health and Human Services; and Julia Francisco, M.P.H., Bureau of Health Promotion, Kansas Department of Health and Environment, for participating in the evaluation process and for their extensive feedback.

To order a copy of this book, contact—

OSH Publications
Mail Stop K-50
Centers for Disease Control and Prevention
4770 Buford Highway NE
Atlanta, GA 30341-3717
Tel.: 770-488-5703 (Press 3 to talk to an information specialist)

For more information on CDC activities
related to tobacco control, visit our Web site:
www.cdc.gov/tobacco

Contents

Executive Summary — 1

Introduction — 5

1. Engage Stakeholders — 15
    The stakeholders in tobacco-use prevention and control — 15
    Why stakeholders are important to an evaluation —16
    The role of stakeholders in an evaluation — 17

2. Describe the Program — 21
    The need for the program — 22
    Goals and objectives — 24
    Program activities — 28
    Program resources — 29
    Stage of development — 30
    Program context — 30
    Logic models — 30
    How to link the program components — 32

3. Focus the Evaluation Design — 37
    Process evaluation — 37
    Outcome evaluation — 39
    Common types of evaluation designs — 42
    Purpose — 44
    Defining the users of evaluation results — 45
    Defining the uses of evaluation results — 46
    Evaluation questions — 46

4. Gather Credible Evidence — 49
    Measuring program outcomes — 49
    Selecting indicators to measure outcomes — 52
    Selecting data sources for indicators — 54
    Suggested data-collection activities for different levels of resources — 57
    Collecting data — 59
    Selecting data-collection methods — 60

5. Justify Conclusions — 67

Analyzing the findings — 67

Interpreting the findings — 68

Sample benchmarks for performance — 68

6. Ensure Use of Evaluation Findings, and Share Lessons Learned — 71

Making recommendations — 71

Sharing the results and the lessons learned from evaluation — 73

Using the information — 74

References — 77

Glossary — 81

Appendices

A: Surveillance and Evaluation Data Resources for Comprehensive Tobacco Control Programs — 87

B: Preventing the Initiation of Tobacco Use Among Young People — 109

C: Promoting Smoking Cessation Among Young People and Adults — 117

D: Evaluation Contracts Checklist — 127

Executive Summary

This document is a "how to" guide for planning and implementing evaluation activities. The manual reflects the priorities of the Centers for Disease Control and Prevention (CDC), Office on Smoking and Health (OSH), for program monitoring and evaluation. The purpose of this manual is to assist state tobacco control program managers and staff in the planning, design, implementation, and use of practical and increasingly comprehensive evaluations of tobacco control efforts. The strategy presented in this manual will aid those responsible for evaluation activities to demonstrate accountability to diverse stakeholders. In this case, accountability includes assessing and documenting the effectiveness of programs, measuring program outcomes, documenting implementation and cost effectiveness, and increasing the impact of programs.

Why evaluate programs to prevent and control tobacco use?

Tobacco use is the leading preventable cause of death and disease in the United States, contributing to more than 430,000 deaths annually.[1] Tobacco control programs are designed ultimately to help reduce disease, disability, and death related to tobacco use. To determine the effectiveness of these programs, one must document and measure both their implementation and their effect. Program evaluation is a tool used to assess the implementation and outcomes of a program, to increase a program's efficiency and impact over time, and to demonstrate accountability.

Program implementation

The task of evaluation encourages us to examine the operations of a program, including which activities take place, who conducts the activities, and who is reached as a result. In addition, evaluation will show how well the program adheres to implementation protocols. Through program evaluation we can determine whether activities are implemented as planned and identify program strengths, weaknesses, and areas for improvement. For example, a smoking cessation program may be very effective for those who complete it, but it may not be attended by many people. Evaluation activities may determine that the location of the program or prospective participants' lack of transportation is an attendance barrier. As a result, program managers can try to increase attendance by moving the class location or meeting times, or by providing free public transportation.

Program effectiveness

The CDC has identified four goals that tobacco control programs should work within to reduce tobacco-related morbidity and mortality:

- Preventing the initiation of tobacco use among young people.
- Promoting quitting among young people and adults.
- Eliminating nonsmokers' exposure to environmental tobacco smoke (ETS).
- Identifying and eliminating the disparities related to tobacco use and its effects among different population groups.

Comprehensive tobacco control programs use multiple strategies to address these goals. Typically, strategies are grouped into three program components: community mobilization, policy and regulatory action, and the strategic use of media. Program evaluation includes documenting the effectiveness of these strategies in meeting program goals.

Program accountability

Program evaluation is a tool with which to demonstrate accountability to program stakeholders (including state and local officials, policymakers, and community leaders) by showing them that a program really does contribute to reduced tobacco use and less exposure to ETS. Evaluation findings can thus be used to show that money is being spent appropriately and effectively and that further funding, increased support, and policy change might lead to even more improved health outcomes. Evaluation helps ensure that only effective approaches are maintained and that resources are not wasted on ineffective programs.

This manual is based on the CDC's *Framework for Program Evaluation in Public Health Practice*[3] and is aligned with the *Healthy People 2010*[4] objectives for the nation, *Best Practices for Comprehensive Tobacco Control Programs*,[2] and other relevant guidelines. This manual is an adaptation of the CDC evaluation framework and is specific to tobacco control and prevention. It is organized into the following six steps:

- Engage stakeholders.
- Describe the program.
- Focus the evaluation and design.
- Gather credible evidence.
- Justify conclusions.
- Ensure use of evaluation findings, and share lessons learned.

Introduction

The health consequences of tobacco use

Tobacco use is the single most preventable cause of death and disease in our society. Annually, in the United States, tobacco use causes more than 430,000 deaths.[1] Direct medical costs related to smoking total at least $50 billion per year;[5] lost productivity adds another $50 billion.[6] Tobacco use is addictive: nearly 70% of smokers want to quit smoking, but only 2.5% are able to quit permanently each year.[7] Most smokers start smoking as adolescents.[8] One in three teenagers who are regular smokers will eventually die of smoking-related causes.[9]

Other tobacco products also have serious health consequences. Use of smokeless tobacco is associated with leukoplakia and oral cancer.[10,11] There is also strong evidence of causal relationships between regular cigar use and cancers of the lungs, larynx, oral cavity, and esophagus.[12] These consequences are of particular concern because in 1999, 15.3% of U.S. high school students smoked cigars and 6.6% used smokeless tobacco.[13]

The risks of tobacco use extend beyond the actual users. Nearly 9 of 10 nonsmoking Americans have been exposed to environmental tobacco smoke (ETS).[14] Exposure to ETS increases nonsmokers' risk for lung cancer and heart disease.[15] Among children, ETS is also associated with serious respiratory problems, including asthma, pneumonia, and bronchitis.[15,16] In addition, scientific evidence now links ETS with sudden infant death syndrome (SIDS) and low birth weight.[15]

How to prevent and control tobacco use

Data from California, Massachusetts, Oregon, Arizona, and a growing number of other states have shown that implementing comprehensive tobacco control programs produces substantial reductions in tobacco use. Comprehensive tobacco control programs seek ultimately to reduce disease, disability, and death related to tobacco use by fulfilling the four CDC program goals:

- Preventing the initiation of tobacco use among young people.
- Promoting quitting among young people and adults.

- Eliminating nonsmokers' exposure to environmental tobacco smoke (ETS).
- Identifying and eliminating the disparities related to tobacco use and its effects among different population groups.

To achieve these goals, CDC recommends that states establish tobacco control programs that are comprehensive, sustainable, and accountable. On the basis of its analyses of comprehensive state tobacco control programs, CDC has identified a number of "best practices" to prevent and control tobacco use.[2] *Best Practices for Comprehensive Tobacco Control Programs*[2] is a guide to help states plan and budget for comprehensive tobacco control programs. *Best Practices* provides a justification for each program element, budget estimates for successful implementation, core resources to assist implementation, and references to scientific literature.

As outlined in *Best Practices*, a comprehensive tobacco control program must include surveillance and evaluation to ensure that tobacco control programs are achieving their goals.[4,17]

What is program evaluation?

Program evaluation is "the systematic collection of information about the activities, characteristics, and outcomes of programs to make judgments about the program, improve program effectiveness, and/or inform decisions about future program development."[18] Program evaluation does not occur in a vacuum and is influenced by real-world constraints. Evaluation should be practical and feasible and must be conducted within the confines of resources, time, and political context. Moreover, evaluation should serve a useful purpose, be conducted in an ethical manner, and produce accurate findings. Evaluation findings should be used to make decisions about program implementation and to improve program effectiveness.

These are some of the questions program evaluation can answer: Is your program making a difference? Is your program effective in reducing tobacco consumption? Can your program be improved? What exactly is your program achieving? Is your program accomplishing what it was intended to accomplish? Was your program implemented as planned? Are you using resources efficiently and effectively? Is your program's performance on par with established standards?

The difference between research and program evaluation

Perhaps the greatest misunderstanding about program evaluation is that it must follow an academic research model. Academic research focuses primarily on testing hypotheses. A key purpose of practical program evaluation is to improve practice. We tend to think of research as requiring a controlled environment or control groups. In tobacco prevention and control, this is seldom realistic. Table 1 shows the principles that distinguish research (conducted, for example, to find the cause of a disease) and evaluation (conducted, for example, to find whether a particular intervention works or whether the program is reaching its intended audience).

Table 1. Distinguishing Principles of Research and Program Evaluation

Concept	Research Principles	Program Evaluation Principles
Planning	**Scientific method** ■ State hypothesis. ■ Collect data. ■ Analyze data. ■ Draw conclusions.	**Framework for program evaluation** ■ Engage stakeholders. ■ Describe the program. ■ Focus the evaluation design. ■ Gather credible evidence. ■ Justify conclusions. ■ Ensure use and share lessons learned.
Decision Making	**Investigator-controlled** ■ Authoritative.	**Stakeholder-controlled** ■ Collaborative.
Standards	**Validity** ■ Internal (accuracy, precision). ■ External (generalizability).	**Repeatability program evaluation standards** ■ Utility. ■ Feasibility. ■ Propriety. ■ Accuracy.
Questions	**Facts** ■ Descriptions. ■ Associations. ■ Effects.	**Values** ■ Merit (i.e., quality). ■ Worth (i.e., value). ■ Significance (i.e., importance).
Design	**Isolate changes and control circumstances** ■ Narrow experimental influences. ■ Ensure stability over time. ■ Minimize context dependence. ■ Treat contextual factors as confounding (e.g., randomization, adjustment, statistical control). ■ Comparison groups are a necessity.	**Incorporate changes and account for circumstances** ■ Expand to see all domains of influence. ■ Encourage flexibility and improvement. ■ Maximize context sensitivity. ■ Treat contextual factors as essential information (e.g., system diagrams, logic models, hierarchical or ecological modeling). ■ Comparison groups are optional (and sometimes harmful).
Data Collection	**Sources** ■ Limited number (accuracy preferred). ■ Sampling strategies are critical. ■ Concern for protecting human subjects. **Indicators/Measures** ■ Quantitative. ■ Qualitative.	**Sources** ■ Multiple (triangulation preferred). ■ Sampling strategies are critical. ■ Concern for protecting human subjects, organizations, and communities. **Indicators/Measures** ■ Mixed methods (qualitative, quantitative, and integrated).

Table 1

Table 1. Distinguishing Principles of Research and Program Evaluation *(continued)*		
Concept	Research Principles	Program Evaluation Principles
Analysis & Synthesis	**Timing** ■ One-time (at the end). **Scope** ■ Focus on specific variables.	**Timing** ■ Ongoing (formative and summative). **Scope** ■ Integrate all data.
Judgments	**Implicit** ■ Attempt to remain value-free.	**Explicit** ■ Examine agreement on values. ■ State precisely whose values are used.
Conclusions	**Attribution** ■ Establish time sequence. ■ Demonstrate plausible mechanisms. ■ Control for confounding. ■ Replicate findings.	**Attribution and contribution** ■ Establish time sequence. ■ Demonstrate plausible mechanisms. ■ Account for alternative explanations. ■ Show similar effects in similar contexts.
Uses	**Disseminate to interested audiences** ■ Content and format varies to maximize comprehension.	**Feedback to stakeholders** ■ Focus on intended uses by intended users. ■ Build capacity. **Disseminate to interested audiences** ■ Content and format varies to maximize comprehension. ■ Emphasis on full disclosure. ■ Requirement for balanced assessment.

Table 1 (continued)

What is surveillance?

Surveillance is the continuous monitoring or routine collection of data on various factors (e.g., behaviors, attitudes, deaths) over a regular interval of time. Surveillance systems have existing resources and infrastructure. Although data gathered by surveillance systems can be useful for evaluation, they serve other purposes besides evaluation. Some surveillance systems (e.g., Current Population Survey [CPS], and state cancer registries) have limited flexibility when it comes to adding questions that a particular program evaluation might like to have answered. Additional examples of surveillance systems include the Behavioral Risk Factor Surveillance System (BRFSS), Youth Tobacco Survey (YTS), and Youth Risk Behavior Survey (YRBS).

The relationship between surveillance and evaluation

Surveillance and *evaluation* are terms that are often used together. However, they are two distinct concepts. It is important to clarify the purposes of surveillance and evaluation.

Evaluation provides tailored information to answer specific questions about a program. Data collection in evaluation is more flexible than in surveillance and may allow program areas to be assessed in greater depth. For example, states can use detailed surveys to evaluate how well a program was implemented and the impact of a program on participants' knowledge, attitudes, and behavior. States can also use qualitative methods (e.g., focus groups, feedback from program participants, and semistructured or open-ended interviews with program participants) to gain insight into the strengths and weaknesses of a particular program activity.

Surveillance and evaluation can and should be conducted simultaneously. To assess tobacco-use prevention and control efforts adequately, states will usually need to supplement surveillance data with data collected to answer specific evaluation questions. States can collect data on, for example, knowledge, attitudes, behaviors, and environmental indicators (e.g., local legislative information, public opinion/poll data, and data on community norms). They can also collect program planning and implementation information to document and measure the effectiveness of a program, including its policy and media efforts.

Why evaluate tobacco control programs?

Data gathered during evaluation enable managers and staff to create the best possible programs, to learn from mistakes, to make modifications as needed, to monitor progress toward program goals, and to judge the success of the program in achieving its short-term, intermediate, and long-term outcomes. Tobacco-use prevention and control programs are designed to promote social and behavioral change and create an environment that reinforces nonsmoking behaviors and supports healthy lifestyles. These changes will lead to reductions in tobacco use and exposure to ETS. Through program evaluation, we can track these changes and, with careful evaluation designs, assess the effectiveness and impact of a particular program, intervention, or strategy (Box 1).

Why evaluate tobacco prevention and control programs?

- To monitor progress toward the program's goals.
- To demonstrate that a particular tobacco control program or activity is effective.
- To determine whether program components are producing the desired effects.
- To permit comparisons among groups, particularly among populations with disproportionately high tobacco use and adverse health effects.
- To justify the need for further funding and support.
- To learn how to improve programs.
- To ensure that only effective programs are maintained and resources are not wasted on ineffective programs.

Box 1

Recognizing the importance of evaluation in public health practice and the need for appropriate methods, the World Health Organization (WHO) established the Working Group on Health Promotion Evaluation. The Working Group prepared a set of conclusions and related recommendations to guide policymakers and practitioners.[19] Recommendations immediately relevant to the evaluation of comprehensive tobacco control programs include—

- Encourage the adoption of participatory approaches to evaluation that provide meaningful opportunities for involvement by all of those with a direct interest in initiatives (programs, policies, and other organized activities).
- Require that a minimum of 10% of the total financial resources for a health promotion initiative be allocated to evaluation.
- Support the use of multiple methods to evaluate health promotion initiatives.
- Support further research into the development of appropriate approaches to evaluating health promotion initiatives.
- Support the establishment of a training and education infrastructure to develop expertise in the evaluation of health promotion initiatives.
- Create and support opportunities for sharing information on evaluation methods used in health promotion through conferences, workshops, networks, and other means.

This manual illustrates how to apply CDC's *Framework for Program Evaluation in Public Health Practice*[3] to the field of tobacco prevention and control. The framework is organized into the following six steps:

- Engage stakeholders.
- Describe the program.
- Focus the evaluation.
- Gather credible evidence.
- Justify conclusions.
- Ensure use of evaluation findings, and share lessons learned.

These six steps must be taken in any evaluation of tobacco prevention and control efforts. The steps are interdependent and not necessarily linear. Looking at Figure 1, you can see that each step builds on the successful completion of earlier steps. Each step in the framework is also associated with standards for "good" evaluation. There are four standards of evaluation that will help you design a good and practical evaluation: utility, feasibility, propriety, and accuracy.[20]

Utility: Does the evaluation have a constructive purpose? Will the evaluation meet the information needs of the various stakeholders? Will the evaluation provide relevant information in a timely manner?

Feasibility: Are the planned evaluation activities realistic? Are resources used prudently? Is the evaluation minimally disruptive to your program?

Propriety: Is the evaluation ethical? Does the evaluation protect the rights of individuals and protect the welfare of those involved?

Accuracy: Will the evaluation produce valid and reliable findings?

How to select a lead evaluator and establish an evaluation team

The evaluation team should include internal program staff, external stakeholders, and possibly consultants or contractors with evaluation expertise. An initial step in the formation of a team is deciding who will be responsible for planning and implementing evaluation activities. At least one program staff person should be selected as the lead evaluator to coordinate program evaluation efforts on behalf of the health department. This lead evaluator should be responsible for evaluation activities, including planning and budgeting for evaluation, developing program objectives, addressing data-collection needs, reporting findings, and working with consultants. The

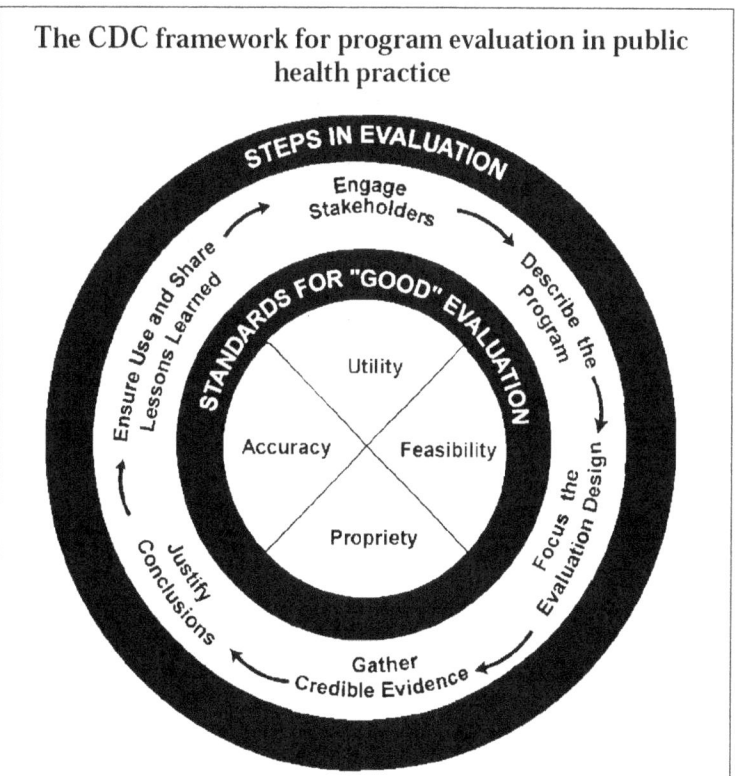

Figure 1

lead evaluator is ultimately responsible for engaging stakeholders, consultants, and other collaborators who bring the skills and interests needed to plan and conduct the evaluation. Although this staff person should have the skills necessary to competently coordinate evaluation activities, if necessary he or she can choose to look elsewhere for technical expertise to design and implement specific evaluation tasks. However, developing in-house evaluation expertise and capacity is a beneficial goal for the health department. See Box 2 for a list of the characteristics of the good evaluator.

Additional evaluation expertise can be found in other programs within the health department, through external partners (e.g., universities, organizations, and companies), from other states' tobacco control programs, and through technical assistance offered by CDC. An additional resource for states includes the CDC's Prevention Research Centers (PRC) program. The PRC program is a national network of 24 academic research centers committed to prevention research and the translation of that research into programs and policies. The centers work with state health departments and members of their communities to develop and evaluate state and local interventions that address the leading causes of death and disability in the nation. Linking university researchers, health agencies, community organizations, and national nonprofit organizations facilitates the translation of promising research findings into practical, innovative, and effective programs. Additional information on the PRCs is available at www.cdc.gov/prc/index.htm.

To supplement the internal evaluation capacity of the health department, you can also use outside consultants as volunteers, advisory panel members, or contractors. External consultants can provide high levels of evaluation expertise from an objective point of view. Important factors to consider when selecting consultants are their level of professional training, experience, and ability to meet your needs. Overall, it is important to find a consultant whose approach to evaluation, background, and training best fits your program's evaluation needs and goals (Box 2). The Evaluation Contracts Checklist presented in Appendix D was designed to help evaluators and clients identify key issues for contracting an evaluation or pieces of an evaluation. Advance agreements on the scope of the evaluation and process can mean the difference between an evaluation's success and failure.

> *A prevention research center in action*
>
> - The West Virginia University Prevention Research Center worked with the American Lung Association and schools and communities in West Virginia and across the United States to develop and evaluate a smoking-cessation program for teenagers called Not On Tobacco (N-O-T).

To generate discussion around evaluation planning and implementation, several states have formed evaluation advisory panels. Advisory panels typically generate input from select local, regional, or national experts otherwise difficult to access. The formation of an evaluation advisory panel will lend additional credibility to your efforts and prove useful in cultivating widespread support for evaluation activities.

In summary, select a lead evaluator who has experience in conducting the type of evaluation you need and a history of evaluating similar programs. In addition, be sure to check all references carefully before you enter into a contract with any consultant. All of the characteristics of a good evaluator listed are important; however, given the value of working with a team, the evaluator's ability to work with a diverse group of stakeholders warrants highlighting. The lead evaluator should be willing and able to draw on community values, traditions, and customs and to work with knowledgeable community members in designing and conducting the evaluation.

Characteristics of a good evaluator

- Has experience in the type of evaluation needed.
- Is comfortable with qualitative and quantitative data sources and analysis.
- Is able to work with a wide variety of stakeholders, including representatives of target populations.
- Can develop innovative approaches to evaluation while considering the realities affecting a program (e.g., a small budget).
- Incorporates evaluation into all program activities.
- Understands both the potential benefits and risks of evaluation.
- Educates program personnel about designing and conducting the evaluation.
- Will give staff the full findings (i.e., will not gloss over or fail to report certain findings for any reason).
- Has strong coordination and organization skills.
- Explains material clearly and patiently.
- Respects all levels of personnel.
- Communicates well with key personnel.
- Exhibits cultural competency.
- Delivers reports and protocols on time.

Box 2

The evaluation team members should clearly define their respective roles. One approach is to develop a written agreement that describes who will conduct the evaluation and assigns specific roles and responsibilities to individual team members. The agreement may either be formal or informal, but it is necessary to clarify 1) the purpose of the evaluation, 2) the potential users of the evaluation findings and plans for dissemination, 3) the way the evaluation will be conducted, 4) the resources available, and 5) protection for human subjects. The agreement should also include a time line and a budget for the evaluation.

1 Engage Stakeholders

The first step in program evaluation is to engage the stakeholders. Stakeholders are people or organizations who are invested in the program, are interested in the results of the evaluation, and have a stake in what will be done with the results of the evaluation. Their needs and interests should be represented throughout the program planning and evaluation process.

The stakeholders in tobacco-use prevention and control

There are three major groups of stakeholders integral to program evaluation:[3]

- Those served or affected by the program, such as patients or clients, advocacy groups, community members, and elected officials.

- Those involved in program operations, such as management, program staff, partners, the funding agency or agencies, and coalition members.

- Primary intended users of the evaluation findings—those in a position to make decisions about the program, such as partners, the funding agency, coalition members and the general public or taxpayers.

If you have been working in tobacco-use prevention and control for a while, you may feel that you already know your stakeholders. However, it is always a good idea to check your assumptions by asking a diverse group of people whom they see as important stakeholders. An inclusive and participatory approach to evaluation includes tapping the unique knowledge of lay people and nonprofessionals from the beginning. In addition, involving a diverse group of stakeholders helps to ground the evaluation in practical reality and better ensures that the information gained through the evaluation benefits all participants.[19]

Possible stakeholders in tobacco prevention and control programs

- Program managers and staff.
- Local, state, and regional coalitions interested in reducing tobacco use.
- Local grantees of tobacco-related funds.
- Local and national partners, such as the American Cancer Society, the Smokeless States Project, the American Lung Association, the American Heart Association, the Centers for Disease Control and Prevention, the American Legacy Foundation, the Substance Abuse and Mental Health Services Administration, and the Robert Wood Johnson Foundation.
- Funding agencies, such as national and state governments.
- State or local health departments and health commissioners.
- State education agencies, schools, and educational groups.
- Universities and educational institutions.
- Local government, state legislators, and state governors.
- Privately owned businesses and business associations.
- Health care systems and the medical community.
- Religious organizations.
- Community organizations.
- Private citizens.
- Program critics.
- State agencies, such as the state department of education and Medicaid.
- Representatives of populations disproportionately affected by tobacco use.
- Law enforcement representatives.

> *A participatory approach to evaluation...*
>
> - Reduces suspicion and fear.
> - Increases awareness and commitment.
> - Allows for differing perspectives.
> - Integrates the knowledge and experiences of diverse stakeholders.
> - Increases the likelihood that evaluation findings will be used.
> - Acknowledges the unique situations of communities.

Why stakeholders are important to an evaluation

Stakeholders are important to program evaluation for several reasons. Considering the perspectives and interests of your various stakeholders will increase the likelihood that your evaluation findings will be accepted and used. Tobacco prevention and control programs rely heavily on partnerships.

Understanding the value systems of your major partners helps maintain these relationships and ensures a useful evaluation. Involving diverse stakeholders will also deepen your understanding of the social and political contexts in which various components of the program operate.

Social and political contexts will likely have implications for the program and the evaluation. Stakeholders bring their own expertise to the table, and involving them in the evaluation process will give you access to a broad range of knowledge, from statistical methods to cultural understandings of tobacco use in a specific population. Stakeholders are much more likely to support the evaluation and act on the evaluation results and recommendations if they are involved in the evaluation process. The presence of stakeholders may also lend credibility to your evaluation. Without stakeholder support, your evaluation may be ignored, criticized, resisted, or even sabotaged.

The role of stakeholders in an evaluation

Stakeholders can be involved in the evaluation at various levels. For example, you may want to include coalition members in an evaluation team and engage them in question development, data collection, and analysis. Or, consider ways to assess your partners' needs and interests in the evaluation, and develop means of keeping them informed of the evaluation's progress and of integrating their ideas into evaluation activities. At a minimum, ensure that the larger network of stakeholders has the opportunity to provide input into designing evaluation questions and is kept informed of the progress of the evaluation. Again, stakeholders are more likely to support the evaluation and act on results and recommendations if they are involved in the evaluation process.

In addition, it can be beneficial to engage your program's critics in the evaluation. In some cases, these critics can help you identify issues around program strategies and evaluation information that could be attacked or discredited, thus helping you strengthen the evaluation process. This information might also help you and others understand the opposition's rationale and could help you engage potential agents of change within the opposition. However, use caution when interacting with the tobacco industry. It is important to understand the motives of the opposition before engaging them in any meaningful way.

> ### Working with stakeholders
>
> - Stakeholders should be consulted and, if appropriate, involved directly, throughout the evaluation process, within time and resource limitations.
> - Stakeholders' interests, expectations, priorities, and commitment to involvement should be assessed at the outset of the evaluation.
> - Communication between stakeholders should be honest and open.
> - Evaluation should be sensitive to the social and cultural environment of the program and its stakeholders.

Engaging diverse stakeholders in the evaluation process is the first step toward a participatory approach to evaluation. A participatory evaluation combines systematic inquiry with the collaboration of diverse stakeholders to meet specific needs and to contend with broad issues of equity and justice.

The Study of Participatory Research in Health Promotion, commissioned by the Royal Society of Canada, attempted to clarify what is meant by a participatory process by providing a working definition and a set of guidelines for use by evaluators and by funding agencies when appraising projects purporting to be participatory.[22] The guidelines emphasize how the normal ways of conducting health research in populations need to adapt to meet the educational, capacity building, and policy expectations of more participatory approaches. Some of the same challenges apply to program evaluation.

✓ Checklist for engaging stakeholders

- Identify stakeholders.
- Identify stakeholder role(s) in evaluation planning and implementation.
- Review the list of stakeholders to ensure all appropriate stakeholders are included.
- Represent individual stakeholders and stakeholder organizations.
- Understand and respect stakeholders' values.
- Create a plan for stakeholder involvement.
- Identify areas for stakeholder input.
- Bring stakeholders together as needed.
- Target key stakeholders for regular participation.
- Ask stakeholders to suggest evaluation questions.

Resources

1. CDC Evaluation Working Group
   www.cdc.gov/eval

2. CDC Prevention Research Centers
   www.cdc.gov/prc/index.htm

3. Health Promotion Evaluation: Recommendations to Policy-Makers: Report of the WHO European Working Group on Health Promotion Evaluation. Copenhagen, Denmark: World Health Organization, Regional Office for Europe; 1998.
   www.who.dk/document/e60706.pdf

4. Green LW, Lewis FM. Measurement and Evaluation in Health Education and Health Promotion. Palo Alto, CA: Mayfield Publishing Company; 1986.

5. Study of Participatory Research in Health Promotion: Review and Recommendations for the Development of Participatory Research in Health Promotion in Canada. Ottawa, Ontario, Canada: Royal Society of Canada; 1995.

6. George MA, Daniel M, Green LW. Appraising and Funding Participatory Research in Health Promotion. The International Quarterly of Community Health Education, Volume: 18 Issue: 2

7. California Tobacco Control Update, August 2000
   www.dhs.cahwnet.gov/tobacco/html/publications.htm

8. Delivering Results: Saving Lives and Saving Dollars Tobacco Prevention and Education in Oregon
   www.ohd.hr.state.or.us/tobacco/arpt2000/welcome.htm

The resources listed here include links to some nongovernmental organizations' Web sites. These sites are provided solely as examples. Links do not constitute an endorsement of these organizations' materials or programs by CDC or the federal government. CDC is not responsible for the content of any individual organization's Web pages found at these links.

Describe the Program

Another early step in evaluation is to develop a clear and succinct description of your program that will clarify the program's purpose, activities, and capacity to decrease tobacco use and improve health. This description is necessary for two reasons:

- To ensure that the stakeholders share the same level of understanding about the program's components, implementation, and intended effects.
- To foster strategic thinking about the program.

In many cases, the process of negotiating with stakeholders to formulate a concise program description will produce benefits long before data are available to measure program effectiveness.[18]

Once you have appropriate stakeholders at the table, you need to make sure that they all have the same knowledge and information about the program and that they view the program from a shared frame of reference. To do so, you will need to describe the program's components and its possible effects clearly. This program description should include the need for the program, its expected effects, the proposed activities of the program, the resources available to conduct the program, the program's stage of development, the social and political context in which the program will be implemented, and a working logic model. (Logic models are discussed in detail beginning on page 30.)

To create change effectively, you need to have clearly linked goals, objectives, and strategies. By looking at your program in this manner you can determine whether an action or event has the potential to cause the desired effect. Doing so may also enable you to identify gaps or missing links between your program's actions and its desired effects.

The need for the program

The description of the need for your program should explain the health problem addressed by the program. In it, you should answer the following questions:

- What is the health problem and its consequences for the state or community?
- What is the size of the problem overall and in various segments of the population?
- What are the determinants of the health problem?
- Who are the target groups?
- What changes or trends are occurring?

The description of the need for your program should include an analysis of the magnitude of tobacco use and related morbidity and mortality in various segments of the population in your state. Do not overlook the economic burden of tobacco use in your state. Analyses of the estimated costs associated with tobacco-related morbidity and mortality will further clarify the need for your program. Smoking Attributable Morbidity, Mortality, & Economic Costs (SAMMEC) software version 3.0 can be used to calculate deaths, years of potential life lost, direct health care costs, indirect mortality costs, and disability costs associated with cigarette smoking. SAMMEC is designed to calculate the health and economic burden of disease from tobacco use at the national and state levels for adults 35 years or older. (Additional information on SAMMEC is in Appendix A.)

Ideally, you should use state or regional data in combination with national data to justify the need for a comprehensive tobacco-use prevention and control program. It is important to identify tobacco-related health disparities among specific population segments or communities when discussing the need for your program. This is a first step in reaching populations disproportionately impacted by tobacco-related morbidity and mortality.

In accordance with *Healthy People 2010*,[4] disparities include but are not limited to differences that occur by gender, race or ethnicity, education or income, sexual orientation, geography, or disability status. Identifying and eliminating the disparities related to tobacco use and its effects among different population groups is the fourth goal of the CDC's National Tobacco

Control Program (NTCP). This goal is unique in that it is both an independent objective and an overarching priority within the other three NTCP goals. For example, a key goal of a state program may be to decrease exposure to ETS. Upon closer examination, the state may find that a particular subgroup or community has a significantly higher prevalence of ETS exposure than the general population. Once this has been established, the state could address the tobacco-related health disparities of this particular subgroup by ensuring the development and implementation of targeted interventions.

To assist you in identifying disparate populations in your state, CDC is in the process of compiling supporting information for the fourth goal. These materials include a logic model, sample objectives, indicators, and potential data sources. The section to follow provides a starting point for the identification of disparate populations in your state. Additional materials will be disseminated by CDC, as available.

Identifying high-risk and historically underserved populations will help program managers, staff, and stakeholders in focusing interventions when state data specific to the health status of diverse communities are not complete. This process requires a working knowledge of the make-up of your state population.

The State Data Center (SDC) Program is one of the Census Bureau's longest and most successful partnerships. It is a cooperative program between the states and the Census Bureau that was created in 1978 to make data available locally to the public through a network of state agencies, universities, libraries, and regional and local governments. The program's mission is to provide easy and efficient access to U.S. Census Bureau data and information through a wide network of lead, coordinating, and affiliate agencies in each state, the District of Columbia, and the outlying areas of American Samoa, Guam, Northern Mariana Islands, Puerto Rico, and the Virgin Islands.

The SDCs are official sources of demographic, economic, and social statistics produced by the Census Bureau. The SDCs make these data accessible to state, regional, local, and tribal governments and to nongovernmental data users at no charge or on a cost-recovery or reimbursable basis, as appropriate. The SDCs also provide training and technical assistance in accessing and using Census Bureau data for research, administration, planning, and decision making by local governments, the business community, and other interested data users. Additional information, including contact information for your state, is available at www.census.gov/sdc/www.

Program managers, staff, and stakeholders are also encouraged to consider available national and state data addressing the health status of specific groups. For example, indicators of tobacco-related disparities include, but are not limited to, prevalence, access to effective and appropriate cessation programs, issues of addiction and relapse, morbidity, mortality, current policies (e.g., policies related to exposure to ETS, youth access, health insurance), and tobacco industry marketing (e.g., targeted advertising and promotions). Other indicators are capacity and infrastructure (e.g., availability of researchers or research data; the availability of appropriate and effective programs, community leadership, organizations, and networks). Sources of data for these indicators include, but are not limited to, national and state surveys, regional or community surveys, case studies, expert panels, and stakeholder panels. The identification of disparate populations is a collaborative process and should involve a diverse group of stakeholders.

Goals and objectives

You should also describe the goals and objectives of your program. To be considered successful, what does your program need to accomplish? The answer to this question depends on what is realistic and achievable given your resources and the maturity and comprehensiveness of the program. Clearly defined objectives are critical to program evaluation because they identify the targets by which you will measure your program's progress.

A *goal* expresses the overall mission or purpose of a program. The goals of a program will guide its development. In tobacco prevention and control, the overarching purpose is to reduce tobacco-related morbidity and mortality. As previously noted, comprehensive tobacco control programs seek to reduce disease, disability, and death related to tobacco use by fulfilling the four CDC program goals:

- Preventing the initiation of tobacco use among young people.
- Promoting quitting among young people and adults.

- Eliminating nonsmokers' exposure to environmental tobacco smoke (ETS).
- Identifying and eliminating the disparities related to tobacco use and its effects among different population groups.

Objectives are statements describing the results to be achieved and the manner in which these results will be achieved. In tobacco control, program objectives should be conceptually linked at the national, state, and local levels. In other words, objectives at the local level should not be selected in isolation, but should be logical extensions of national and state objectives.

The specific objectives outlined in *Healthy People 2010*[4] are a starting point for tobacco control efforts. CDC encourages NTCP partners to use the objectives outlined in *Healthy People 2010* as an initial guide for focusing state activities. The complete list and a discussion of *Healthy People 2010* tobacco objectives are available online at www.health.gov/healthypeople.

Good objectives are specific and measurable. Well-written and clearly defined objectives are important because they–

- Set program priorities.
- Aid in monitoring progress toward achieving goals.
- Set targets for accountability.

A well-written and clearly defined objective is SMART: **S**pecific, **M**easurable, **A**chievable and **A**mbitious, **R**elevant, and **T**ime bound.

Specific:	It identifies a specific event or action that will take place.
Measurable:	It quantifies the amount of change to be achieved.
Achievable and **A**mbitious:	It is realistic given available resources and plans for implementation, yet challenging enough to accelerate program efforts.
Relevant:	It is logical and relates to the program's goals.
Time-bound:	It specifies a time by which the objective will be achieved.

Here is an example of a SMART objective:

In state X, increase the percentage of adult nonsmokers who report they have not been exposed to cigarette smoke in the prior 7 days from 40% in 2001 to 50% in 2010.

- The objective is *specific* because it identifies a defined event: adult nonsmokers will not be exposed to cigarette smoke.

- The objective is *measurable* because it specifies a baseline value and the quantity of change the intervention is designed to achieve: from 40% to 50%. It would be worthwhile to note whether there is already a data source for the objective.

- The objective is *achievable* because it is realistic given the 10-year time frame and *ambitious* because achieving the goal would be a significant accomplishment.

- The objective is *relevant* because it relates to the elimination of exposure to ETS.

- The objective is *time-bound* because it provides a specified time by which the objective will be achieved (from 2001 to 2010).

There are two general types of objectives: process and outcome. *Process objectives* describe program activities. They specify actions to be taken and are useful in measuring program implementation. Outcome objectives are the intended results of program activities. They quantify anticipated program effects by specifying "the amount of change expected for a given health problem/condition for a specified population within a given time frame."[23] Outcome objectives are often divided into short-term, intermediate, and long-term objectives. They generally state "who will achieve how much of which outcome by when." "Who" is typically stated as a population; "how much" as a percentage or target amount; and "by when" as a month, or year(s), or period after the program begins.[24,25,26]

Objectives must logically link to each other. For one long-term outcome objective, there may be several intermediate outcome objectives. Similarly, there may be a number of process objectives for each short-term outcome objective. Below are examples of outcome and process objectives specific to the goal of eliminating exposure to ETS. These examples assume that baseline data collected to identify tobacco-related disparities among population groups indicated that African American adults and children were disproportionately burdened by tobacco-related morbidity and mortality. Complete sets of example objectives for two goal areas—preventing the initiation of tobacco use among young people and promoting smoking cessation amoung young people and adults—can be found in Appendices B and C.

Program goal
Eliminate exposure to environmental tobacco smoke in state A.

Sample long-term objectives for eliminating exposure to ETS
- Decrease the percentage of adult nonsmoking African Americans exposed to ETS at work from X% in 2002 to Y% in 2007.
- Increase the percentage of African Americans younger than age 18 who, during the previous 7 days, have not been in the same room with someone who was smoking from X% in 2002 to Y% in 2007.

Sample intermediate objectives
- Increase the percentage of African American adults who are employed at work sites with a formal policy that prohibits smoking at the workplace from X% in 2002 to Y% in 2005.
- Increase the percentage of African American homes that have household smoking bans from X% in 2002 to Y% in 2005.
- Increase the percentage of African American adults who report asking someone not to smoke around them in order to avoid exposure to their tobacco smoke from X% in 2002 to Y% in 2005.

Sample short-term objectives
- Increase the percentage of adults who believe that breathing secondhand smoke is harmful to them from X % in 2002 to Y % in 2003.
- Increase the percentage of adults who believe smoking should not be allowed in workplaces from X % in 2002 to Y % in 2003.
- Increase the percentage of adults who believe that breathing secondhand smoke is harmful to children from X % in 2002 to Y % in 2003.

Sample process objectives

- By March 2002, design a media campaign about the health effects of ETS and the importance of smoke-free homes and automobiles, with tailored messages for African American families.

- By April 2002, negotiate placement of at least two billboards on the harmful effects of ETS in each of the eight major African American communities in the state.

- By August 2002, publish at least three antitobacco newspaper articles on ETS in at least two community newspapers in the state.

- By May 2002, develop model voluntary smoke-free policies tailored to work sites with African American employees.

- By July 2002, distribute sample voluntary smoke-free policies to at least 50 % of work sites in communities with African American populations of more than 5,000.

SMART objectives should be rooted in well-planned program activities. Like program objectives, program activities should be linked at the local, state, and national levels to maximize their effect.

Program activities

Program activities describe what the program is actually doing to affect the health problem. For example, possible tobacco control activities to reduce youth smoking rates might include counter-marketing, retailer enforcement, and school-based prevention programs. It is important to describe the different activities, determine how they relate to each other and to the program's goals, and identify the different steps or actions expected to occur. Program activities are often specified in a series of process objectives.

National Tobacco Control Program (NTCP) Matrix

COMPONENTS	GOALS			
	Prevent Initiation Among Youth	Promote Quitting Among Young People and Adults	Eliminate Exposure to ETS	Identify and Eliminate Disparities Among Population Groups
Community Interventions				
Counter-Marketing				
Policy/ Legislation				
Surveillance/ Evaluation	X	X	X	X

Figure 2

States often describe their tobacco control efforts using a program framework. A program framework such as the National Tobacco Control Program (NTCP) Matrix (Figure 2) clearly outlines program components and links them to evidence-based strategies and goals. The NTCP Matrix can apply to planning and implementing state and local activities. Regardless of which goal you are focusing on, *surveillance and evaluation* is a necessary component.

States may choose to organize their programs according to funding categories for budget-planning purposes. CDC's *Best Practices for Comprehensive Tobacco Control Programs* describes nine components of comprehensive tobacco control programs.[2] You may want to consider these when describing your program:

- Community programs to reduce tobacco use.
- Chronic disease programs to reduce the burden of tobacco-related diseases.
- School programs to prevent or delay the onset of smoking during the school year.
- Enforcement of tobacco control policies to enhance their efficacy.
- Statewide programs to increase the capacity of local programs and expand their reach.
- Counter-marketing efforts to counter pro-tobacco influences and increase pro-health messages and influences.
- Cessation programs to assist youth and adult smokers to quit.
- Surveillance and evaluation activities to monitor and document implementation and achievement for stakeholders.
- Administration and management to facilitate collaboration and coordination among public health program managers, policymakers, and other state agencies.

In many instances, program components highlighted in the NTCP Matrix and *Best Practices* overlap. It is worthwhile to consider both approaches prior to describing program activities.

Program resources

Resources necessary to conduct a tobacco control program include money, staff, time, materials, and equipment. Program evaluation activities often include accountability for resources to funding agencies and stakeholders. Therefore, you should clearly identify the resources you need to administer the program.

Stage of development

Stage of development describes the maturity of a program. The stage of your program's development will influence the type of evaluation you want to do and the outcomes you will measure. The CDC evaluation framework recognizes at least three stages of program development: planning, implementation, and effects.

Program context

Program context refers to the environment in which a program exists. Because external factors can influence your tobacco control program, you should be aware of and understand them. Factors that can influence program context include politics, funding, interagency support, competing organizations, competing interests, social and environmental conditions, and history of leadership (of the program, agency, and past collaborations). In tobacco prevention and control, program context includes the influences of the tobacco industry, such as the price of tobacco products, taxes, advertising and promotions, political contributions, and the state of the tobacco economy. Also included are tobacco-related lawsuits, the level of enforcement of tobacco-related laws, and even the amount of publicity surrounding violations or penalties.

Logic models

Logic models link program inputs (i.e., resources) and activities to program outcomes (Figure 3). Logic models are tools that can be used to 1) identify the short-term, intermediate, and long-term outcomes for your program; 2) link those outcomes to each other and to program activities; 3) select indicators to measure, depending on the stage of your program's development; and 4) explain to decision makers why it may take time before you are able to demonstrate long-term outcomes associated with your program.

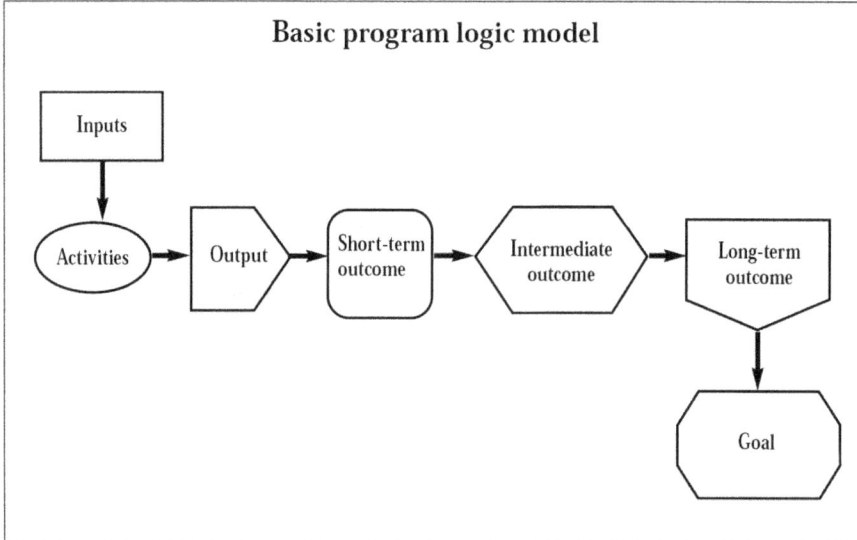

Figure 3

Inputs are the various resources that go into a program. Inputs for a tobacco control program include—

- Direct and in-kind funding.
- Staffing.
- Partner organizations.
- Equipment.
- Materials.

Activities are the actual events that take place as part of the program. The following are examples of the activities of a tobacco control program targeting a Latino population:

- Develop a media plan to educate and inform the selected Latino population about the dangers of ETS.
- Assess the cultural appropriateness of the media campaign.
- Fund and establish 15 local and 17 regional coalitions to work on ETS issues.
- Conduct a media campaign targeting the Latino population.
- Develop coalitions that work with schools and day care centers to educate children and young people about the hazardous health effects of ETS exposure.
- Develop coalitions to encourage restaurant owners to adopt smoke-free policies.

Outputs are the direct products of program activities. The following are some examples:

- A written plan for media campaigns tailored to specific populations.
- The number of smokers enrolled in cessation courses.
- The number of ETS posters placed in stores and buses.
- The number of young people signed up to join advocacy groups.

Outcomes are the intended effects of the program.

Short-term outcomes are the immediate effects of a program and often focus on the knowledge, attitudes, and skills gained by a target audience. The following are some examples:

- Increased public exposure to information about the dangers of ETS and the purpose of smoking bans.

> *Other names for a logic model*
> - Theory of change.
> - Model of change.
> - Theoretical underpinning.
> - Causal chain.
> - Weight-of-evidence model.
> - Roadmap.
> - Conceptual map.
> - Blueprint.
> - Rationale.
> - Program theory.
> - Program hypothesis.

- Increased knowledge among school and day care center personnel about the health effects of ETS exposure on children and young people.
- A more positive attitude toward smoke-free policies among business owners.
- Increased understanding by parents about the effects of ETS in the home.

Intermediate outcomes include behavior change, normative change, and changes in policies. The following are some examples:

- Adoption of clean indoor air policies.
- Institution of voluntary bans on smoking in schools and day care centers, restaurants, and work places.
- An increase in the percentage of adults (with children in the home) who implement household smoking restrictions.

Long-term outcomes take years to achieve. The following are some examples:

- Decreases in the prevalence of tobacco use.
- Reduced exposure to ETS.
- Decreased tobacco-related morbidity and mortality among targeted populations.
- Reduced overall tobacco-related morbidity and mortality.

> *Logic model components*
>
> - **Inputs:** Resources that go into the program.
> - **Activities:** Actual events or actions that take place.
> - **Outputs:** Direct products of program activities, often measured in terms of the amount of work accomplished (e.g., the number of clients served or sessions held).
> - **Outcomes:** Impact of the program; the sequence of effects triggered by the program, often expressed in terms of short-term, intermediate, and long-term outcomes.
> - **Goal:** Overall mission or purpose of the program.

How to link the program components

When drafting a logic model, first determine your goal, then assess program inputs (resources) and decide on activities. Once you have selected your program's activities, ask "If we do this, then what will happen?" For example,

- If we develop a Request For Applications (RFA) to fund coalitions to address a targeted population's exposure to ETS, then we can establish coalitions.
- If we establish the coalitions, then they will implement a tobacco prevention program to address targeted populations' exposure to ETS.
- If the coalitions implement ETS prevention counter-marketing programs that target specific populations, then these populations will be exposed to messages explaining the health hazards of ETS.

- If targeted populations are exposed to information about the health hazards of ETS, then at least some of that population will believe ETS is harmful to themselves and to children.

- If targeted populations believe ETS is harmful, then they may be motivated to change their smoking behaviors.

- If targeted populations are motivated to change their smoking behaviors, then they may change their smoking behaviors and support bans on smoking.

- If targeted populations change their smoking behaviors and support bans on smoking, then they will be exposed to less ETS.

- If targeted populations are exposed to less ETS, then they will have less morbidity and mortality attributable to tobacco use.

After you have decided on the various components of your logic model, arrange them in a logical order, starting at the left-hand side and moving to the right (Figure 3). Examine the model carefully. Does each step logically relate to the other? Are there missing steps that disrupt the logic of the model? Once the model is implemented, can you use it to assess whether your program is doing what it needs to do to implement change? It is important to remember that logic models change over time with improvements to the program, shifting resources, and innovations in the science of tobacco-use prevention and control.

Logic models can be broad or specific. They can be linked to one another to express how programs connect at the national, state, and local levels. In addition, you could prepare a set of logic models to represent diverse aspects of the program: an overall state program, multi-strategy efforts to address one of the four goal areas, or a specific program strategy within a goal area such as a media campaign to promote smoke-free homes. Figures 4 and 5 are two examples of logic models representing different levels of detail. The logic model in Figure 4 is general and depicts the logic underlying the NTCP. Figure 5 is specific to eliminating exposure to ETS. Logic models for the other goal areas are in Appendices B and C.

In summary, drafting logic models can be challenging but worthwhile. Logic models can help you determine whether your program activities logically lead to the desired outcome. A visual description of the program helps ensure that all the stakeholders understand the program's purpose, the resources it will need, the activities it will conduct, and its capacity to effect change. Logic models are useful starting places for forming questions to be answered through the evaluation. Finally, collaborating with stakeholders to create logic models is an effective way to engage them in the evaluation and to generate support for your program.

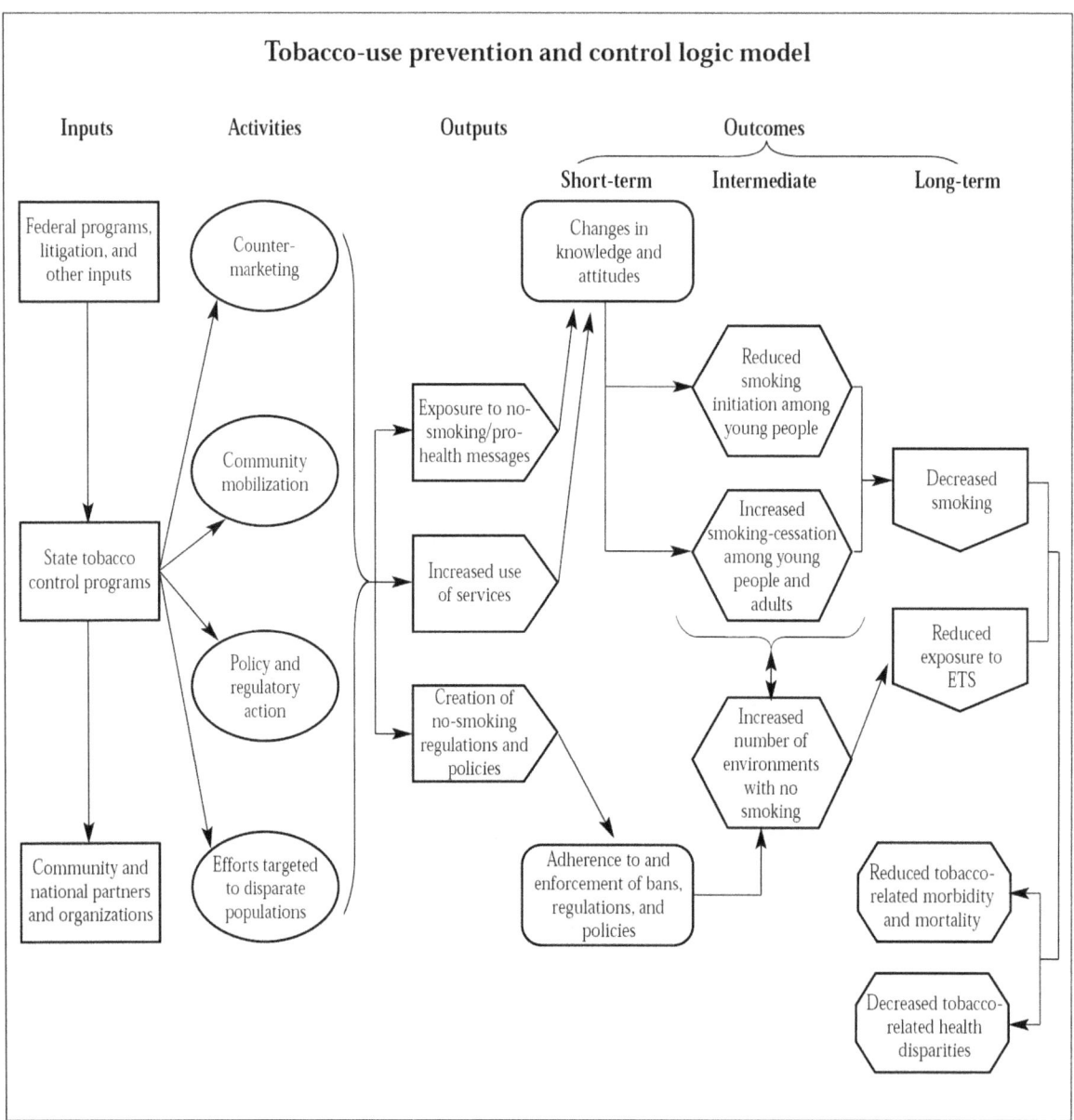

Figure 4

2. Describe the Program

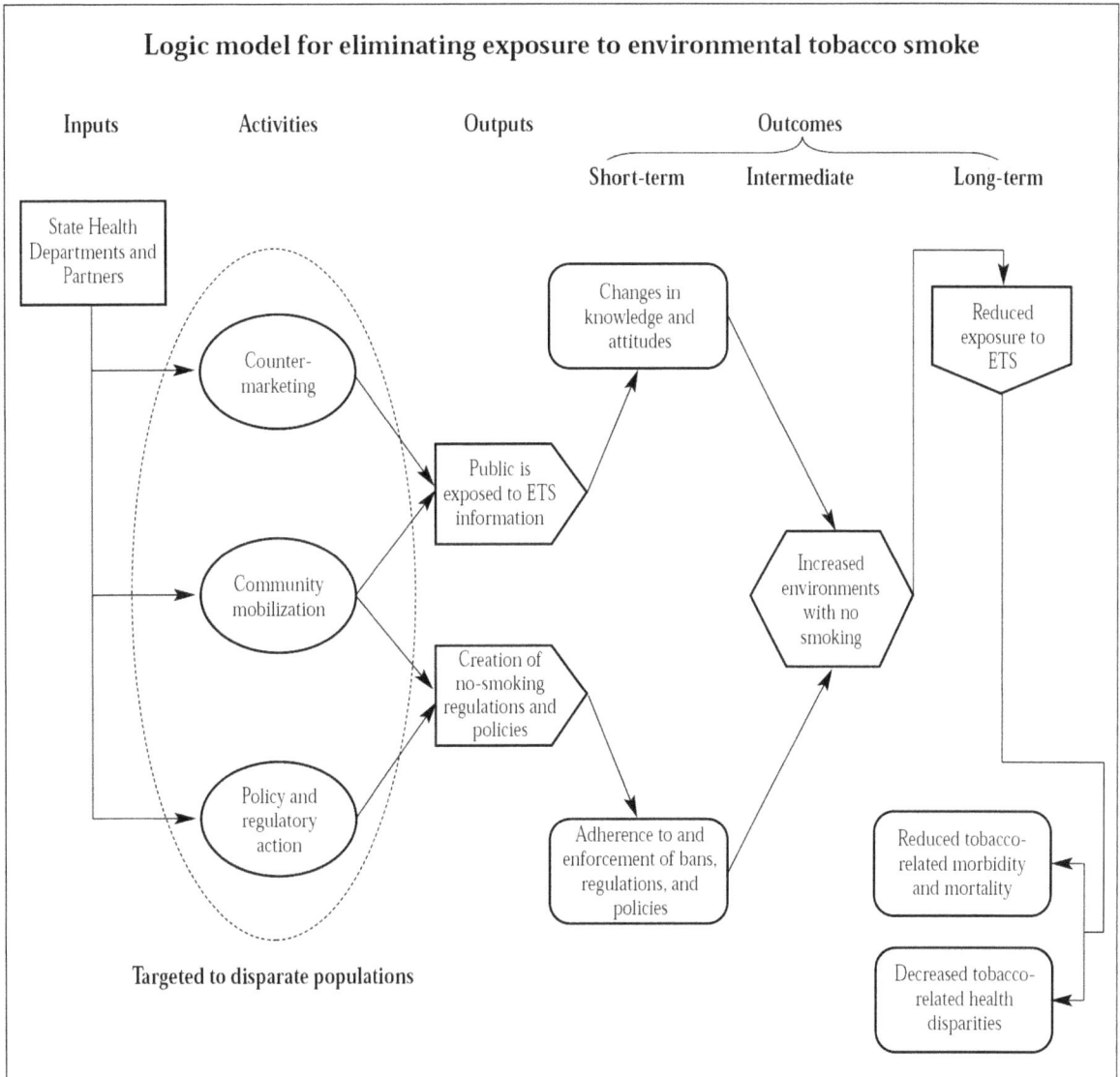

Figure 5

✓ Checklist for describing the program

- Document the need for the program.
- Document program resources.
- Note the program's stage of development.
- Explain the program context.
- List and describe program activities.
- State program goals and objectives.
- Prepare a logic model.

Resources

1. CDC Evaluation Working Group
   www.cdc.gov/eval

2. U.S. Census Bureau State Data Center Program
   www.census.gov/sdc/www

3. *Healthy People 2010*
   www.health.gov/healthypeople

Focus the Evaluation Design

Now that you and your stakeholders have a clear understanding of your program, your evaluation team will need to focus the evaluation. The evaluation team must decide the purpose of the evaluation and the questions it wants answered. A typical approach to evaluation in public health is to design data-collection systems that monitor progress toward meeting a program's process and outcome objectives. Initially, you may not be able to collect baseline data and track progress toward all of your objectives. However, it is important to remember that baseline data are valuable for planning and evaluation and should be collected if possible. Rather than trying to answer every question that various stakeholders may pose, the evaluation team should focus on those it determines to be the most important questions about your program. A focused evaluation requires "advance planning about where the evaluation is headed and what steps will be taken to get there."[3]

Having a focused evaluation makes it easier to conduct a quality evaluation. The design should outline which questions you are investigating, the process you will follow, what will be measured, what methods will be used, who will perform each activity (including analysis and interpretation), what you will do with the information once it is collected, and how the results will be disseminated.

Process evaluation

Process evaluations are used to document how well a program has been implemented; they are conducted periodically throughout the duration of a program. This type of evaluation is used to examine the operations of a program, including which activities are taking place, who is conducting the activities, and who is reached through the activities. Process evaluations assess whether inputs or resources have been allocated or mobilized and whether activities are being implemented as planned. They identify program strengths, weaknesses, and areas that need improvement. Following are examples of the type of tangible program indicators measured by process evaluation:

- The locale where services or programs are provided (e.g., rural, urban).
- The number of people receiving services.
- The economic status and racial/ethnic background of people receiving services.
- The quality of services.
- The actual events that occur while the services are delivered.
- The amount of money the project is using.
- The direct and in-kind funding for services.
- The staffing for services or programs.
- The number of activities and meetings.
- The number of training sessions conducted.

A process evaluation of a counter-marketing campaign to reduce the number of young people who start smoking might answer questions such as these:

- Has a workgroup been formed and is it meeting regularly?
- Are any key individuals or organizations missing from the workgroup?
- Was the counter-marketing campaign designed on schedule?
- Have the campaign products (posters, billboard, radio and television spots) been pretested?
- Are project activities being implemented on schedule?
- What barriers have been encountered?
- Who is the campaign's target audience and how well are they being reached?
- How many advertisements are actually running? When and where?
- Where are the posters/billboards located?
- What is the estimated number of people who see or hear the advertisements?
- How might the action plan be improved on the basis of evaluation findings?

Process evaluations can also assess issues related to program services. For example, they can determine the—

- Availability and use of tobacco-use treatment services.
- Implementation of smoking prevention programs in schools and the community.
- Accessibility of resource centers and materials.
- Amount of technical support and training provided to grantees or staff.
- Amount of technical support and training needed by grantees or staff.
- Number of calls to a quitline.
- Use of the quitline by various racial/ethnic groups.
- Extent of insurance coverage for tobacco-use treatment.
- Percentage of primary care physicians who give advice and assistance on quitting.
- Number of health care systems that have implemented tobacco-use reminder systems.
- Use of Food and Drug Administration (FDA)-approved medications by Medicaid recipients.

These are straightforward questions; monitoring them throughout the duration of your program ensures that the project is implemented as planned and is reaching the intended audience.

Outcome evaluation

Outcome evaluations are used to assess the impact of a program on the stated short-term, intermediate, and long-term objectives. This type of evaluation assesses what has occurred because of the program and whether the program has achieved its outcome objectives. Outcome evaluations should be conducted only when the program is mature enough to produce the intended outcome.

Outcome evaluations can measure the following:

- Changes in people's attitude toward, and beliefs about, tobacco, their awareness of and support for your program, and their perception of how well tobacco-related policy is being enforced.

- Changes in intended and actual tobacco-related behaviors.
- Changes in the environment, such as changes in public and private policies, in formal and informal enforcement of minors' access and nonsmoking regulations, and in the influence of pro-tobacco forces.
- Changes in populations, such as in the average age at which people begin smoking, per capita consumption of cigarettes, and smoking prevalence.
- Changes in trends in morbidity and mortality.

In this manual, program outcomes are divided into three levels: short-term, intermediate, and long-term. Decisions as to whether a particular outcome is short-term, intermediate, or long-term depend on the purpose of the program and the time needed for the change to occur. For example, there are no strict guidelines for whether a policy change is a short-term or an intermediate outcome; it could also be thought of as a process measure.

Similarly, changes in per capita consumption could be considered an intermediate or a long-term outcome. Whether outcomes are considered short- or long-term is less important than whether sound logic underlies the program. Do the short-term outcomes lead logically to the intermediate outcomes? Do the intermediate outcomes lead logically to the long-term outcomes? Is adequate time allowed to reasonably expect to see an effect?

Short-term outcomes are the immediate or early results of the program. Short-term outcomes may be changes in knowledge, attitudes, and skills. For example, in a program with the goal of reducing children's exposure to ETS, a short-term outcome might be having parents who smoke show increased knowledge about the danger of smoking around children.

Intermediate outcomes reflect further progress in reaching a program goal. Intermediate outcomes link short-term outcomes with long-term outcomes. Intermediate outcomes may be changes in individual behaviors, social norms, or the environment. An intermediate outcome in the program described in the previous paragraph might be that the parents no longer smoke around their children.

Long-term outcomes reflect the ultimate goal of the program. The long-term outcome in the previously described program would be decreased morbidity from children's exposure to ETS.

For a tobacco control program with the goal of reducing the number of young people who start smoking through a counter-marketing campaign, an outcome evaluation might examine whether the targeted young people exhibit—

- Increased knowledge and awareness of the dangers of smoking (short-term outcome).

- Changes in tobacco-related attitudes and beliefs (intermediate outcome).

- Changes in tobacco-related behavior (long-term outcome).

- Changes in smoking rates and age of initiation (long-term outcome).

- Changes in morbidity and mortality (long-term outcome).

Comparing tobacco-related data among states and between one state and the nation as a whole are common and important ways to evaluate tobacco control programs. Another option is to compare data from different—but relevant—sources. For example, you could make comparisons using indicators from the YTS, the BRFSS tobacco module, PRAMS, and a survey of adult tobacco use. Comparing your data with national data and other states' data will help you to establish realistic objectives for your program and meaningful benchmarks for progress. States can also compare their progress with that of states with a similar investment in tobacco control, or they can contrast their results (outcomes) with the results that could be expected if their program were similar to those of states with a larger investment in tobacco control.

Comparison data are also useful for measuring indicators in anticipation of new or expanding programs. For example, noting a "lack of change" in key indicators over time prior to program implementation helps demonstrate the need for your program and highlights the comparative progress of states with comprehensive tobacco control programs already in place. A lack of change in indicators may continue for several years and is useful as a justification for greater investment in evidence-based, well-funded, and more comprehensive programs. There are many opportunities for between-state comparisons and trend analysis, which can be highlighted with time-series analyses. The tobacco questions on many of the larger surveillance systems have not changed in several years, so you can make comparisons with other states and over time, using specific indicators. Program managers are encouraged to collaborate with state epidemiologists, BRFSS coordinators, and statisticians to make state and national comparisons an important component of your evaluation.

Common types of evaluation designs

The field of health promotion is under increasing pressure to demonstrate that programs are worthwhile, effective, and efficient. During the last 2 decades, knowledge and understanding about how to evaluate complex programs have increased significantly. The appropriateness of the evaluation design is a primary concern. The evaluation design ought to accommodate the complexity of program activities and meet the needs of diverse stakeholders. As a result, states are often encouraged to use multiple methods to evaluate program efforts. However, "the use of randomized control trials to evaluate health promotion initiatives is, in most cases, inappropriate, misleading, and unnecessarily expensive."[19]

Three general types of evaluation designs are commonly recognized: experimental, quasi-experimental, and observational. Evaluations using experimental designs use random assignment to compare the effect of an intervention on one or more groups with effect on an equivalent group or groups that did not receive the intervention. For example, an evaluation team could select a group of similar schools, then randomly assign some schools to receive a tobacco-use prevention curriculum and other schools to serve as control schools. All schools have the same chance of being selected as an intervention or control school. Because of the "random assignment," you reduce the chances that the control and intervention schools vary in any way that could influence differences in program outcomes. This allows you to attribute change in outcomes to your program. For example, if the students in the intervention schools delayed smoking onset longer than students in the control schools, you could attribute the success to your program.

Sometimes in community settings it is hard, or even unethical, to have a true control group. One solution is to offer the program to the control group after data for the evaluation have been collected. Another option is to use a quasi-experimental design. These designs make comparisons between nonequivalent groups and do not involve random assignment to intervention and control groups. An example would be to assess adults' beliefs about the harmful effects of ETS in two communities, then conduct a media campaign in one of the communities. After the campaign, you would reassess the adults and expect to find a higher percentage of adults believing ETS is harmful in the community that received the media campaign. Critics could argue that other differences between the two communities caused the changes in beliefs, so it is important to document that the intervention and comparison groups are similar on key factors such as population demographics and related current or historical events.

Observational designs are also used in program evaluation. These include, but are not limited to, longitudinal, cross-sectional surveys and case studies. Periodic cross-sectional surveys (e.g., the YTS or BRFSS) can inform your evaluation. Case studies may be particularly appropriate for assessing changes in tobacco control capacity in disparate population groups. Case studies are often applicable when the program is unique, when an existing program is used in a different setting, when you are assessing a unique outcome, or when an environment is especially unpredictable. Case studies can also allow for an exploration of community characteristics and how these may influence program implementation as well as the identification of barriers to and facilitators of change. One resource on case studies is *Using Case Studies To Do Evaluation*, by the California Department of Health Services' Tobacco Control Section (www.dhs.cahwnet.gov/ps/cdic/ccb/TCS/documents/ProgramEvaluation.pdf). This guide can help evaluators determine whether and how to use a case study approach.

Given the widespread visibility of antitobacco messages and overlapping program components, traditional evaluation designs (experimental and quasi-experimental) have proven difficult to implement and hard to maintain. Some tobacco control program outcomes are often detectable only after several years.

Therefore, before choosing an experimental or quasi-experimental design for your evaluation, consider the appropriateness and feasibility of less traditional designs (e.g., simple before-after [pretest-posttest] or posttest-only designs). Depending on your program's objectives and the intended use(s) for the evaluation findings, these designs may be more suitable for measuring progress toward achieving program goals. And these designs often cost less and require less time. Keep in mind, however, that saving time and money should not be the main criterion when selecting an evaluation design. It is important to choose a design that will measure what you need to measure and that will meet both your immediate and long-term needs.

A *goal-based evaluation model* uses predetermined program goals as the standards for evaluation, thus holding the program accountable to prior expectations. In such cases, evaluation planning focuses on the activities, outputs, and short-term, intermediate, and long-term outcomes outlined in a program logic model to direct measurement activities. One advantage of this evaluation model is that the evaluation team has flexibility and can adapt evaluation strategies if notable changes occur in the inputs and activities of the program. In the early stages of your program, progress toward objectives can be measured to document achievement and demonstrate accountability.

The design you select influences the timing of data collection, how you analyze the data, and the types of conclusions you can make from your findings. A collaborative approach to focusing the evaluation provides a practical way to better ensure the appropriateness and utility of your evaluation design.

Purpose

You should articulate the purposes of your evaluation. These may be to improve the program, assess program effectiveness, or demonstrate accountability for resources. The purposes will reflect the stage of development of your program. With a new program, you will probably want to conduct a process evaluation to help improve the program. With a mature program, you will probably want to conduct an outcome evaluation to assess your program's effectiveness and to demonstrate that it is making productive use of resources.

Improving the program

Program evaluation can identify areas in the program that need improvement. For example, a smoking-cessation program may be effective, but it may not be attracting or retaining many participants. By conducting a process evaluation you may discover why. For example, the program may be at an inconvenient location, or participants may not have access to transportation or child care. Cost may be a barrier. As a result, program coordinators may attempt to increase attendance by moving the location of the class, providing free public transportation, working with purchasers and insurers to increase coverage for programs, or switching to a telephone cessation help-line to increase access.

Assessing the program's effectiveness

Program evaluation can measure how effective your program is at progressing toward the desired outcomes. For example, evaluation can assess whether a school-based tobacco prevention program is increasing students' knowledge about the dangers of tobacco, or whether a cessation program is increasing the duration or permanency of participants' attempts to quit smoking. Information about the effectiveness of a program can be used to make decisions about the continuation, refinement, or expansion of the program.

Demonstrating productive use of resources

Program managers are typically accountable to funders and various stakeholders, including government officials and policymakers. Program managers must justify how and where their funds are spent. Evaluation results can be used to demonstrate that a program is functioning as planned, achieving its objectives, worth the cost, or making an important contribution to health.

Defining the users of evaluation results

The evaluation team must also consider who will use the evaluation results. Those users need to be identified and given the opportunity to provide input into the design of the evaluation. Support from the intended users will increase the likelihood that they will use the evaluation results. Users of evaluation findings differ from the larger network of program stakeholders in that the information needs of intended users will determine how you focus the evaluation.

Defining the uses of evaluation results

How your results will be used depends on the purpose and intended users of the evaluation. You need a plan for each piece of information collected. Consider also why you are collecting it and what you are going to do with it. In tobacco control and prevention, evaluation information may be used, for example,

- To identify areas of the program that need improvement.
- To decide how to allocate resources.
- To document the level of success in achieving objectives.
- To assess community needs.
- To mobilize community support.
- To redistribute or expand the locations where the intervention is carried out.
- To improve the content of the program's materials.
- To focus program resources on a specific population.

Evaluation questions

A focused evaluation gathers information for a specific purpose or use. Evaluation questions need to be discussed with and agreed upon by the stakeholders. After you have identified the evaluation users, you must determine what is important to them and design your evaluation questions to meet their needs. Because the questions your evaluation team and stakeholders agree on will affect the methods you use to gather data, you must decide which questions to ask before you choose your methods.

Besides having a specific purpose and use, your evaluation should also reflect the stage of your program's development. For example, you must decide whether you are conducting an outcome evaluation, a process evaluation, or both. Process evaluations and outcome evaluations require different designs and collect different types of data. Think about the stage of your program's development in making these decisions. If you have a well-established program, you may wish to evaluate changes in intermediate or long-term outcomes. However, the evaluation team should determine which outcomes are the most important to evaluate at each stage of program development. Decisions about the evaluation questions and outcomes you plan to measure should be made by the evaluation team in collaboration with key stakeholders.

> ✓ **Checklist for focusing the evaluation design**
>
> - Define the purpose(s) of your evaluation.
> - Identify the use(s) of the evaluation results.
> - Formulate the questions the evaluation will answer.
> - Distinguish evaluation from research questions.
> - Review evaluation questions with stakeholders, program managers, and program staff.
> - Include process and outcome evaluation.
> - Review options for the evaluation design.
> - Consider a goal-based evaluation model.
> - Make sure that the evaluation design fits the evaluation questions.
> - Collect baseline data.
> - Plan how to compare your data with those of other states and with national data.
> - Consider local or regional comparisons, or both.
> - Seek technical expertise or review.
> - Document the need for the program.
> - Document program resources.
> - Note the program's stage of development.
> - Explain the program context.
> - List and describe program activities.
> - State program goals and objectives.
> - Prepare a logic model.

Resources

1. CDC Evaluation Working Group
   www.cdc.gov/eval

2. Using Case Studies to do Program Evaluation
   www.dhs.cahwnet.gov/ps/cdic/ccb/TCS/html/
   Evaluation_Resources.htm

3. Local Program Evaluation Planning Guide
   www.dhs.cahwnet.gov/ps/cdic/ccb/TCS/html/
   Evaluation_Resources.htm

4. CDC. Strategies for reducing exposure to environmental tobacco smoke, increasing tobacco-use cessation, and reducing initiation in communities and health-care systems. A report on recommendations of the Task Force on Community Preventive Services. *MMWR* 2000;49(No. RR-12).
   www.cdc.gov/tobacco/research_data/environmental/
   rr4912.pdf

5. CDC. Decline in cigarette consumption following implementation of a comprehensive tobacco prevention and education program—Oregon, 1996–1998. *MMWR* 1999;48:140–3.
   www.cdc.gov/tobacco/research_data/interventions/
   mm4807.pdf

6. CDC. Declines in lung cancer rates—California, 1988–1997. *MMWR* 2000;49:1066–70.
   www.cdc.gov/tobacco/research_data/health_consequences/
   ccmm4947.pdf

7. Lois Biener, Jeffrey E Harris, and William Hamilton. Impact of the Massachusetts tobacco control programme: population based trend analysis. *BMJ* 2000; 321:351–4.
   www.bmj.com

The resources listed here include links to some nongovernmental organizations' Web sites. These sites are provided solely as examples. Links do not constitute an endorsement of these organizations' materials or programs by CDC or the federal government. CDC is not responsible for the content of any individual organization's Web pages found at these links.

4 Gather Credible Evidence

Measuring program outcomes

Now that you have written measurable objectives, developed a logic model, and selected your evaluation questions, you can refine the outcomes you want to measure in your evaluation. Although you selected outcomes to prepare your logic model, during evaluation many tobacco control programs expand their set of outcomes for each goal area.

When choosing outcomes to measure, keep in mind the purpose, users, and intended uses of the evaluation. In addition, the outcomes you choose should be relevant, important, and discrete. Although it may be tempting to evaluate only the long-term outcomes of your program, monitoring short-term and intermediate outcomes is also important so you can relate changes in health outcomes to program activities or identify gaps in the program. Moreover, demonstrating short-term impact may help justify continued or additional funding. Measuring the implementation of program activities is also important to ensure that the program is functioning as it should.

On the basis of the ETS logic model shown on page 35 (Figure 5), here are some example outcomes you may choose to measure (stratified by process or outcome level):

Long-term outcomes
- Reduced exposure to ETS.

Intermediate outcomes
- Increased percentage of smoke-free homes.
- Increased percentage of smoke-free private cars.
- New legislation restricting or prohibiting smoking in enclosed public places.
- Increased percentage of workplaces with voluntary bans restricting or prohibiting smoking.

- Increased percentage of public places with nonsmoking policies.
- Increased percentage of restaurants with nonsmoking policies.
- Increased adherence to and enforcement of nonsmoking policies.

Short-term outcomes

- Increased knowledge and awareness about ETS.
- Increased public support for smoke-free public places, workplaces, and schools.
- Increased public exposure to information about ETS.
- Education of policymakers, legislators, workplace managers and owners, and school officials about the harmful effects of ETS exposure.

In process evaluation, the *outcome* is really an *output*. *Outputs* are the direct products of program activities, often measured in terms of the amount of work accomplished, such as the number of clients served or sessions held.

Outputs

- A counter-marketing campaign against ETS has been designed.
- A counter-marketing campaign against ETS has been implemented.
- Model voluntary smoke-free policies have been developed.
- Model smoke-free work-site policies have been distributed.

Before choosing outputs and outcomes to measure, you should first ask yourself these three key questions:

- Is it reasonable to believe the program can influence the outcome, even though it cannot control it?
- Would measuring the outcome show program successes or pinpoint and address problems or shortcomings?
- Would the program's stakeholders accept the outcome or output as a valid result of program activities?

Once you have selected a set of outputs and outcomes to measure, you should ask yourself these questions:

- Do program activities and outputs and short-term, intermediate, and long-term outcomes logically relate to each other?

- Do these relationships reflect the logic of the program—the sequence of influences and changes that program inputs, activities, and outputs are intended to set in motion?

- Do the longer-term outcomes represent meaningful benefits or changes in participants' status, condition, or quality of life?

- Have you considered possible negative outcomes of your program?

The outcomes you choose to measure should be—

- Relevant to the goal and objectives of your program.

- Important to achieve if your program is to attain its objectives.

- Indicative of meaningful changes.

- Influenced by your program.

- Realistic about the scope of influence of your program.

- Useful in identifying both problems and successes of your program.

- Effective in representing the changes or benefits attributable to your program.

As discussed earlier, an evaluation should be focused, have a specific purpose and use, and reflect the program's stage of development. For example, you must prepare to conduct both a process evaluation and an outcome evaluation, as appropriate. Process evaluations and outcome evaluations use different types of data. If you have a well-established program, it may be appropriate to expect changes in intermediate or long-term outcomes. The outputs and outcomes you include in the evaluation should reflect important dimensions of the program at each stage of development. In addition, select outputs and outcomes that will be most informative given the purpose(s) of your evaluation. Identifying and measuring outputs and outcomes can provide the information to fully assess and understand the impact of program efforts and make appropriate program decisions.[19]

Selecting indicators to measure outcomes

Once you have determined the outcomes you want to measure, you need to select indicators. *Indicators* are specific, observable, and measurable characteristics or changes that show the progress a program is making toward achieving a specified outcome.[27] For example, the percentage of adult nonsmokers who report they have not been exposed to cigarette smoke in the previous 7 days is an indicator that can be used to measure the long-term outcome of "decreased exposure of adult nonsmokers to ETS."

Indicators must be relevant to identified focus areas and questions. Be sure that the cost of collecting data on the indicators is within the evaluation budget, and check the source and availability of expected data. Evaluation staff must decide 1) which data collection, management, and analysis strategies are most appropriate for each indicator, and 2) whether needed technical assistance is available and affordable.

To establish indicators for each outcome, you should review selected outcomes and identify "specific, observable accomplishment(s) or change(s) that will tell you whether the outcome has been achieved."[27] Keep the following tips in mind when selecting your indicators:

- There should be at least one indicator for each outcome.
- The indicator must be focused and must measure an important dimension of the outcome.
- The indicator must be clear and specific in terms of what it will measure.
- The change measured by the indicator should represent progress that the program has made toward achieving the outcome.

Commonly used indicators include—

- Participation rates.
- Attitudes.
- Individual behavior.
- Community norms.
- Policies.
- Health status.

Indicators specific to tobacco prevention and control programs include—

- The number of clean indoor air ordinances that have been passed during a given period.
- The proportion of a targeted population group who report having smoked in the last 30 days.
- The percentage of health insurance companies that reimburse for cessation services.

Table 2 provides examples of outcomes, outputs, indicators, and data sources for programs to eliminate exposure to ETS. The indicators are used to document change over time and measure progress toward objectives. Appendix B has examples for the goal of preventing initiation of tobacco use among young people, and Appendix C has examples for the goal of promoting quitting among young people and adults.

Table 2. Example Outcomes, Outputs, Indicators, and Data Sources for the Goal of Eliminating Exposure to Environmental Tobacco Smoke (ETS)

Long-Term Outcomes	Long-Term Indicators	Data Sources*
Decreased exposure of adult nonsmokers to ETS.	■ Percentage of adult nonsmokers who report they have not been exposed to cigarette smoke during the previous 7 days. ■ Percentage of adults who report they are never exposed to cigarette smoke in restaurants. ■ Percentage of adults who report they are not exposed to cigarette smoke at work during a typical work day.	■ Adult Tobacco Survey.
Decreased exposure of young people to ETS.	■ Percentage of young people who report they have not been in the same room as someone smoking in the previous 7 days. ■ Percentage of young people who report they have not been in a car with someone who was smoking in the previous 7 days. ■ Percentage of mothers who report their baby is never in a room with someone who is smoking.	■ Youth Tobacco Survey. ■ Pregnancy Risk Assessment Monitoring System.

Intermediate Outcomes	Intermediate Indicators	Data Sources*
Increased percentage of smoke-free homes and cars.	■ Percentage of adults who report smoking is not allowed in their home. ■ Percentage of adults who report smoking is not allowed in the family car.	■ Adult Tobacco Survey. ■ State surveys.
Increased percentage of workplaces with restrictions or prohibitions on smoking.	■ Percentage of workplaces with policies that prohibit or restrict smoking. ■ Percentage of adults employed at work sites with formal policies that prohibit smoking.	■ Behavioral Risk Factor Surveillance System (Optional Module). ■ State or local policy tracking.
Increased percentage of enclosed public places and restaurants with restrictions on smoking.	■ Percentage of counties with clean air ordinances. ■ Percentage of restaurants that prohibit smoking.	■ State legislative tracking. ■ Local policy tracking.
Increased enforcement of no-smoking laws.	■ Percentage of schools, workplaces, and public places that comply with smoke-free policies or regulations. ■ Percentage of adults who report asking someone not to smoke around them.	■ Site-specific surveys. ■ Adult Tobacco Survey.

Table 2
* For more information on data sources, see Appendix A.

Table 2. Example Outcomes, Outputs, Indicators, and Data Sources for the Goal of Eliminating Exposure to Environmental Tobacco Smoke (ETS)

Short-Term Outcomes	Short-Term Indicators	Data Sources*
Increased awareness of, and exposure to, messages about the hazards of ETS.	■ Percentage of adults who recall the content of an ETS media campaign (which includes brochures, posters, presentations).	■ State surveys.
Increased knowledge and improved attitudes and skills related to ETS.	■ Percentage of adults who believe breathing secondhand smoke is bad for them. ■ Percentage of adults who believe smoking around children is harmful. ■ Percentage of young people who believe breathing secondhand smoke is bad for them. ■ Percentage of young people who believe smoking around children is harmful.	■ Youth Tobacco Survey. ■ Adult Tobacco Survey.
Increased public support for no-smoking policies.	■ Percentage of people who report that they support smoke-free policies. ■ Percentage of people who believe smoking should not be allowed in restaurants, schools, workplaces, and other enclosed public places.	■ Adult Tobacco Survey.
Process Outputs	**Process Indicators**	**Data Sources***
Increased number of smoke-free homes and private cars.	■ A media campaign under way about the negative health effects of ETS.	■ Media materials.
Increased number of smoke-free workplaces.	■ The number of local coalitions that report they distributed examples of smoke-free workplace policies to at least 50% of the manufacturing plants in their area.	■ State progress reports. ■ Copy of the model smoke-free policy.
Increased public support for smoke-free environments.	■ The number of news stories on ETS in major newspapers. ■ The number of news stories on ETS in Spanish newspapers.	■ Media tracking.

Table 2 (continued)
* For more information on data sources, see Appendix A.

Selecting data sources for indicators

Now that you have determined the outcomes you want to measure and the indicators you will use to measure progress toward those outcomes, you need to select the data sources you will use to gather information on your indicators. Sources of data fall into three categories: people, documents, and observations. Box 3 lists possible sources of information for evaluations within these categories.

When choosing data sources, pick those that meet your data needs. Try to avoid choosing a data source that may be familiar or popular but does not necessarily answer your questions. Keep in mind that budget issues alone should not drive your evaluation planning efforts. Consider the following questions:

- What do you need to know?
- When do you need the data?

- How often do you need the data?
- Will the data be compared with similar data from elsewhere?
- Is credibility of the data an issue?
- How much money do you have to spend?

In evaluating tobacco-use prevention and control programs, you have the option of using existing data systems or building new ones customized to your program's components. Some existing data sources include—

- Behavioral Risk Factor Surveillance System (BRFSS).
- Youth Risk Behavior System (YRBS).
- Pregnancy Risk Assessment Monitoring System (PRAMS).
- Cancer registries.
- Vital statistics.
- National Health Interview Survey (NHIS).
- Youth Tobacco Survey (YTS).
- Adult Tobacco Survey (ATS).
- School Health Policies and Programs Study (SHPPS).

To ensure that these data sources meet your evaluation needs, you may need to modify them. If you use an existing surveillance system to inform aspects of your evaluation, you might want to add state-specific questions or expand the sample size. Expanding the sample size allows for more stable estimates and possible sub-state estimates. Likewise, to produce much-needed data, you may want to invest in oversampling disparate populations.

Sources of information[3]

People
- Clients, program participants, nonparticipants.
- Staff, program managers, administrators.
- Partner agency staff.
- General public.
- Community leaders or key members of a community.
- Funders.
- Critics or skeptics.
- Representatives of advocacy groups.
- Elected officials, legislators, policymakers.
- Local and state health officials.

Observations
- Meetings, special events or activities, job performance.
- Service encounters.

Documents
- Grant proposals, newsletters, press releases.
- Meeting minutes, administrative records.
- Registration or enrollment forms.
- Publicity materials, quarterly reports.
- Publications, journal articles, poster presentations.
- Previous evaluation reports.
- Needs assessments.
- Surveillance summaries.
- Database records.
- Records held by funders or collaborators.
- Web pages.
- Graphs, maps, charts, photographs, videotapes.

Box 3

Keep in mind that, although large ongoing surveillance systems have the advantages of collecting data routinely and having existing resources and infrastructure, some of them (e.g., Current Population Survey [CPS]) have little flexibility with regard to the questions asked in the survey. Therefore, it is difficult (sometimes impossible) to use these systems to collect the special data you need for your evaluation. In contrast, surveys such as YTS, BRFSS, or PRAMS are flexible with regard to the questions asked: you can supplement their questions with your questions to get the data you need. However, the drawback to these surveys is that they are conducted only occasionally, and usually they require an expenditure of funds or other resources.

If the existing data systems cannot answer your evaluation questions, you will need to build a new data system or adopt a system that is not already in your state.

Examples of new data systems:

- State or local policy tracking systems or site-specific surveys (such as those monitoring compliance with the Synar Amendment, and work-site, restaurant, or day-care-center surveys).
- Key informant surveys.
- Health systems and clinical settings surveys.
- Media tracking surveys.
- Systems that monitor pro-tobacco activities (including advertising, event sponsorship, promotional items, discounts).
- Systems that monitor program activities (such as local program monitoring).
- Systems that track sales data.
- Systems that monitor the use of services (e.g., cessation services, education programs, quitlines).

Examples of useful systems that may not yet be in your state:

- School Health Education Profiles (SHEP).
- School Tobacco Survey (STS) (which includes the Lead Health Educator Survey and School Principal Survey).

Suggested data-collection activities for different levels of resources

In general, the purpose of evaluation—rather than the amount of available resources—should determine data-collection strategies. However, we are including the following information as a general guide to help you plan your evaluation using the resources that you have available.

The variation in available resources across states ranges from low to high levels and necessitates a variation in the evaluation activity. As resources increase, investment in key evaluation activities should also increase. In Table 3, we suggest evaluation activities for low, medium, and high levels of resources. However, not all programs should strictly follow this guide because the needs of an evaluation will vary not only with the amount of resources available, but with the intended use of the evaluation data. For example, although only limited resources may be available, evaluation of a program that is primarily focused on funding local activities should include regional or local data on both outcome and process measures.

Table 3. Evaluation Activities You Can Accomplish with Low, Medium, and High Levels of Resources

Sample evaluation activities	Resources		
	With a low level of resources, we suggest	With a medium level of resources, we suggest	With a high level of resources, we suggest
■ Improving your state's infrastructure* for surveillance and evaluation.	Improving *state competency*[†] and *capacity*[‡] to conduct evaluation.	Improving *local competency*[†] to conduct evaluation.	Improving *local capacity*[‡] to conduct evaluation.
■ Using or improving existing data systems for program evaluation.	*Using* existing national and state surveys and data collection systems.	*Improving* existing national and state surveys or data collection systems.	*Further improving* national or state surveys and data-collection systems.
■ Creating new data systems.	Creating and conducting a *state* survey to collect *state* data.	Creating and conducting *regional* surveys to collect *regional* data.	Creating and conducting *local* surveys to collect *local* data.

Table 3
* *Infrastructure:* All the components necessary to conduct evaluation (e.g., experienced staff, adequate funding).
† *Competency:* Staff with the knowledge and experience needed to conduct surveillance and evaluation.
‡ *Capacity:* The resources (e.g., competent staff, appropriate data-collection systems) to conduct evaluation.

Infrastructure

To enhance your program's internal capacity to coordinate and direct evaluation activities, program staff should develop competency in evaluation planning and implementation. Competency also includes having partnerships and in-kind resources within your agency to support program evaluation. You should dedicate staff time for a lead evaluator or evaluation coordinator. As your resources increase and activities expand to the local level, you should develop similar competencies and capacity at that level.

Existing data systems

At a minimum, states should use data from national surveys and state data-collection systems (e.g., BRFSS, YRBS, PRAMS, YTS, Legislative Tracking, NTCP Chronicle). National data systems provide comparison outcome and some process measures for state activities. Comparison data from national surveys and other data-collection systems can be used to evaluate activities across states and to document any lack of change that can be used to justify additional tobacco program funding. By working with system representatives, you can include additional tobacco-related measures on state data-collection instruments and increase the amount and type of data collected on regional and local measures. For example, tobacco control representatives are encouraged to build a partnership with the state BRFSS coordinator to include optional modules or state-added questions on the state BRFSS.

Some state data are easily accessible via the State Tobacco Activities Tracking and Evaluation (STATE) System (www2.cdc.gov/nccdphp/osh/state). The STATE System is the first on-line compilation of state-based tobacco information from many different data sources; it allows the user to view summary information on tobacco use in all 50 states and the District of Columbia. The STATE System contains up-to-date and historical data on the prevalence of tobacco use, tobacco control laws, the health impact and costs of tobacco use, and tobacco agriculture and manufacturing.

New data systems

We strongly encourage states to develop and implement new data-collection systems such as a youth tobacco survey, an adult tobacco survey, subpopulation prevalence surveys, community capacity and infrastructure assessments, a health care provider survey, a media tracking survey, and local policy tracking, as appropriate. New data systems can be developed specifically to provide process and outcome measures for focused or unique program activities. Some states have implemented comparable systems that provide comparison data across certain states. These systems can be designed to provide data at the state or sub-state (e.g., health region, county) levels.

Appendix A describes the different types of national, state, and topic-specific tobacco-related data sources. It also includes a description of the source, tobacco indicators, sampling frame, methodology, years completed, and contact information. (An Internet address is provided for most national data sources.) In the "comments" section is a description of the past use of the data source, advantages, disadvantages, and other details. Many of these data sources provide general and category-specific measures that assess changes in social norms at individual and community levels. You should choose a data source that will provide reliable and credible information about the outcome. You can also use more than one data source for a specific indicator, because multiple data sources will provide a more comprehensive view of your program. Although the data sources listed in Appendix A are almost all quantitative, qualitative data from focus groups, feedback from program participants, and semistructured or open-ended interviews with program participants or key informants are also important sources of information for an evaluation.

Collecting data

Once you have specified the outcomes you want to measure, selected indicators, reviewed existing sources of data, and determined which resources can be devoted to data collection, it is time to collect your data. The data you gather will be used to assess the effectiveness of your program and help you make decisions about your program. Therefore, data collection must produce informative, useful, and credible results. The quality and quantity of data, the collection method used, and the timing of the data collection are all factors that contribute to the credibility of the evidence that you gather in your evaluation. Keep in mind that you may not need to implement annual surveys for some information needs.

For example, community assessments of capacity and infrastructure may only need to be administered every 5 years. And periodic sampling of subpopulations for tobacco use patterns may need to be done only every 2 to 3 years and possibly aggregated for analysis.

Selecting data-collection methods

It is important that the data-collection methods be the most appropriate for measuring the outcomes and indicators you have selected. Some methods are geared toward collecting qualitative data, and others toward collecting quantitative data. Some methods are more appropriate for specific audiences or resource considerations. The methods used must give adequate consideration to the evaluation purpose, the intended users, and what will be viewed as credible evidence.

When choosing a method, think about the following:

The purpose of the evaluation: Which method seems most appropriate for your purpose and the questions that you want to answer?

The users of the evaluation: Will the method allow you to gather information that can be analyzed and presented in a way that will be seen as credible by your intended audience? Will they want standardized quantitative information from a data source such as the Adult Tobacco Survey, or descriptive, narrative information from focus groups, or both?

The respondents from whom you will collect the data: Where and how can respondents best be reached? What is culturally appropriate? For example, is conducting a phone interview or personal, door-to-door interview more appropriate for certain population groups?

The resources available (time, money, volunteers, travel expenses, supplies): Which method(s) can you afford and manage well? What is feasible? Will your evaluation be completed in time for the next legislative session or prior to the end of the school year? Consider your own abilities and time. Do you have an evaluation background or will you have to hire an evaluator? Do program funds and relevant policies allow you to hire external evaluators?

The degree of intrusiveness—interruptions to the program or participants: Will the method disrupt the program or be seen as intrusive by the respondents? Also consider issues of confidentiality, if the information that you are seeking is sensitive.

Type of information: Do you want representative information that applies to all participants (standardized information such as that from a survey, structured interview, or observation checklist that will be comparable nationally and across states)? Or, do you want to examine the range and diversity of experiences, or tell an in-depth story of particular people or programs (e.g., descriptive data as from a case study)?

The advantages and disadvantages of each method: What are the key strengths and weaknesses in each? Consider issues such as time and respondent burden, cost, necessary infrastructure, access to sites and records, and overall level of complexity. What is the most appropriate for your evaluation needs?

Mixed data-collection methods refers to the collection of both quantitative and qualitative data. Mixed methods can be used *sequentially*, when one method is used to prepare for the use of another, or *simultaneously*, when both methods are used in parallel. An example of sequential use of mixed methods is when focus groups (qualitative) are used to develop a survey instrument (quantitative), and then personal interviews (qualitative) are conducted to investigate issues that arose during coding or interpretation of survey data. An example of simultaneous use of mixed methods would be using personal interviews to verify the response validity of a quantitative survey.

Different methods reveal different aspects of the program. For example—

- You might conduct a ***group assessment*** at the end of a school-based tobacco control program to hear the group's viewpoint, as well as ***individual student interviews*** to get a range of opinions.

- You might conduct a ***survey*** of all legislators in a state to gauge their interest in managed care support of cessation services and products, and you might also ***interview*** certain legislators individually to question them in greater detail.

- You might conduct a ***focus group*** with community leaders to assess their attitudes regarding tobacco industry support of cultural and community activities. You might follow the focus group with ***individual structured*** or ***semi-structured interviews*** with the same participants.

Using mixed methods increases the cross-checks on different subsets of findings and generates increased stakeholder confidence in the overall findings. In addition, combining methods provides a way to triangulate findings, which maximizes the strengths and minimizes the limitations of each method. Using mixed methods enables you to validate your findings, enhance reliability, and build a more thorough evaluation for improving program effectiveness.[28]

Quality of data

A quality evaluation produces data that are reliable, valid, and informative. An evaluation is reliable to the extent that it repeatedly produces the same results, and it is valid if it measures what it is intended to measure. The advantage of using existing data sources such as the YTS, BRFSS, YRBS, or PRAMS is that they have been pretested and designed to produce valid and reliable data. If you are designing your own evaluation tools, you should be aware of the factors that influence data quality:

- The design of the data-collection instrument and how questions are worded.
- The data-collection procedures.
- Training of data collectors.
- The selection of data sources.
- How the data are coded.
- Data management.
- Routine error checking as part of data quality control.

Quantity of data

You will also need to determine the amount of data you want to collect during the evaluation. Your study must have a certain minimum quantity of data to detect a specified change produced by your program. In general, detecting small amounts of change requires larger sample sizes. For example, detecting a 5% increase would require a larger sample size than detecting a 10% increase. If you use tobacco data sources such as the YTS, the sample size has already been determined. If you are designing your own evaluation tool, you will need the help of a statistician to determine an adequate sample size.

When assessing the quantity of data you need to collect (often expressed as sample size), you will also need to consider the level of detail and the types of comparisons you hope to make. You

4. Gather Credible Evidence

will also need to determine the jurisdictional level for which you are gathering the data (e.g., state, county, region, congressional district). Counties often appreciate and want county-level estimates; however, this usually means larger sample sizes and more expense.

The next step is choosing a data-collection method. Although it is practical to use or adapt data-collection methods that have been pretested and evaluated for validity and reliability, the methods you choose must be able to answer the questions you want answered. Again, do not settle on a particular method because it is easy, familiar, or popular—the methods should be appropriate to the outcomes you want to measure. Examples of data-collection methods are surveys, interviews, observation, document analysis, focus groups, and case studies.

The most widely used data-collection methods in tobacco prevention and control are surveys, such as the Youth Tobacco Survey. Other methods used include tracking policy changes, running focus groups to test antitobacco counter-marketing messages, reviewing vital statistics for deaths attributed to smoking, and conducting Synar Amendment inspections. For more information on specific data-collection systems, see Appendix A.

You will need to outline procedures to follow when collecting the evaluation data. Consider these issues:

- When will you collect the data? You will need to determine when (and at what intervals) it is most appropriate to collect the information. If you are measuring whether your objectives have been met, your objectives will provide guidance as to when to collect certain data. If you are evaluating specific program interventions such as a smoking-cessation program, you might want to obtain information from participants before they begin the program, upon completion of the program, and several months after the program. If you are assessing the effects of a counter-marketing campaign, you might want to assess tobacco-related knowledge, attitudes, and behaviors among your target audience before and after the campaign.

- Who will be considered a participant in the evaluation? Are you targeting a relatively specific group (African American young people), or are you assessing trends among a more general population (all young people, grades 6–12)?

- Are you going to collect data from all participants or a sample? Many tobacco control programs are community-based, and surveying a sample of the population participating in such programs is appropriate. However, if you have a small number of participants (such as students exposed to a tobacco curriculum in two schools), you may want to survey all the participants.

- How will the information be collected? Will the information be collected by telephone, by mail, or through interviews? How will the information be computerized?

- Who will collect the information? Are those collecting the data trained and trained consistently? Will the data collectors uniformly gather and record information? Your data collectors will need to be trained to ensure that they all collect information in the same way and without introducing bias. Preferably, interviewers should be trained together and by the same person.

- How will the security and confidentiality of the information be maintained? It is important to ensure the privacy and confidentiality of the evaluation participants. You can do this by collecting information anonymously and making sure you keep data stored in a locked and secure place.

- Do you need approval from an institutional review board (IRB) before collecting the data? What will be your informed consent procedures?

The answers to some of these questions depend on your evaluation questions and the design you select to answer those questions. If you mainly want to monitor progress in meeting your objectives (e.g., assess the proportion of work sites with smoke-free policies), you may not need a particular evaluation design beyond monitoring the work sites that go smoke-free. If, however, you want to attribute the change to your program, you would want to use an experimental or quasi-experimental evaluation design.

✓ Checklist for gathering credible evidence

- Prepare to collect process and outcome data.
- Confirm the outcomes are logically linked to program activities.
- Confirm that outcomes are logically linked at the national, state, and local levels.
- Address a continuum of outcomes (short-term, intermediate, and long-term).
- Link outcomes to indicators and data sources.
- Identify at least one indicator for each outcome.
- Determine if you need to create a new data-collection system.
- Pilot test new instruments to identify and/or control sources of error.
- Consider adding evaluation questions to already existing surveillance systems.
- Consider a mixed-method approach to data collection.
- Take into account available resources.
- Consider issues of timing for data collection and reporting needs.

Resources

1. CDC Evaluation Working Group
   www.cdc.gov/eval

2. State Tobacco Activities Tracking and Evaluation (STATE) System
   www2.cdc.gov/nccdphp/osh/state

The resources listed here include links to some nongovernmental organizations' Web sites. These sites are provided solely as examples. Links do not constitute an endorsement of these organizations' materials or programs by CDC or the federal government. CDC is not responsible for the content of any individual organization's Web pages found at these links.

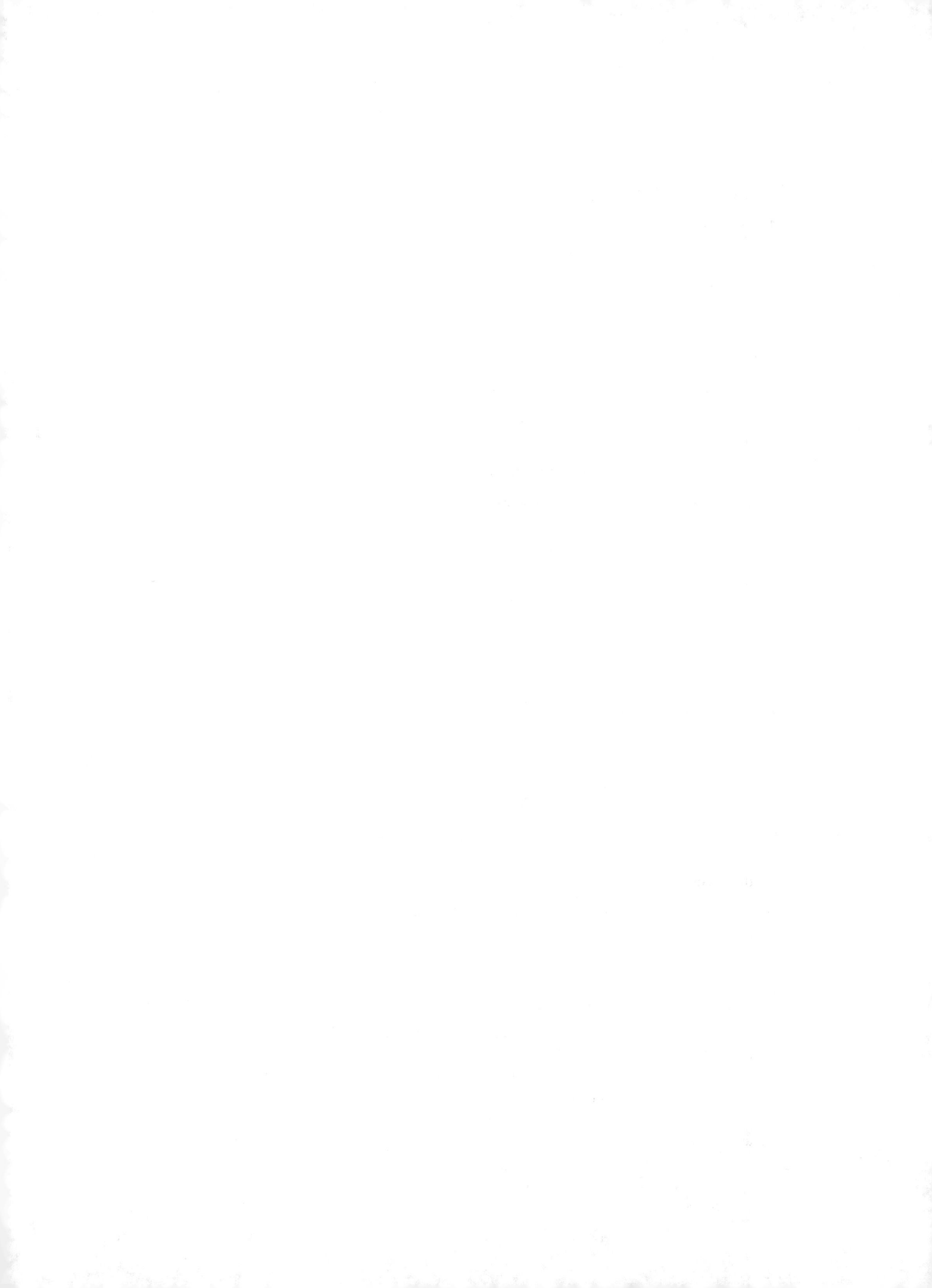

Justify Conclusions

The next step in program evaluation is to prepare the data for the intended use(s) of the evaluation. Whether your evaluation is conducted to show program effectiveness, help improve the program, or demonstrate accountability, you will need to analyze and interpret your findings.

Analyzing the findings

Data analysis is the process of organizing and classifying the information you have collected, tabulating it, analyzing it, comparing the results with other appropriate information, and presenting the results in an easily understandable manner. There are five steps in data analysis:

1. Enter the data into a database and check for errors. If you are using a surveillance system such as BRFSS or PRAMS, the data have already been checked, entered, and tabulated by those conducting the survey. If you are collecting data with your own instrument, you will need 1) to select the computer program you will use to enter and analyze the data, and 2) to determine who will enter, check, tabulate, and analyze the data.

2. Tabulate the data. The data need to be tabulated to provide information (such as a number or percentage) for each indicator. Some basic calculations include determining—

    - The number of participants.
    - The number of participants achieving the desired outcome.
    - The percentage of participants achieving the desired outcome.

3. Analyze and stratify your data by various demographic variables of interest, such as participants' race, sex, age, income level, or geographic location.

4. Make comparisons. Use statistical tests to show differences between comparison and intervention groups, between

geographic areas, or between the pre-intervention and post-intervention status of the target population.

5. Present your data in a clear and understandable form. To interpret your findings and make your recommendations, you must ensure that your results are easy to understand and clearly presented. Data can be presented in tables, bar charts, pie charts, line graphs, and maps.

Interpreting the findings

After analyzing your findings, the next step is to examine your results and determine what they actually say about the program. The purpose of the evaluation, the social and political context of your program, and the needs of the stakeholders are all issues to be considered in relation to your results.

Sample benchmarks for performance

To measure your progress within the national context of tobacco prevention and control, you need to compare your data with national data and with the data of other states. *Healthy People 2010* objectives provide a starting point for performance measurement from a national perspective. However, a clear set of standards for assessing a tobacco prevention and control program's success in attaining short-term and intermediate outcomes has not been developed. Therefore, it is important to develop a set of standards against which you will measure your progress. Possible standards include—

- Needs of participants.
- Community values, expectations, and norms.
- Program mission and objectives.
- Program protocols and procedures.
- Changes in selected indicators over time.
- Performance by similar programs.
- Performance by a control or comparison group.
- Resource efficiency.
- Mandates, policies, regulations, and laws.
- Judgments of participants, experts, and funders.
- Institutional goals.
- Social equity.
- Human rights.

Tips to remember when interpreting your findings[29]

- Interpret evaluation results with the goals of your tobacco control program in mind.
- Keep your audience in mind when preparing the report. What do they need and want to know?
- Consider the limitations of the evaluation:
  - Possible biases.
  - Validity of results.
  - Reliability of results.
  - Generalizability of results.
- Are there alternative explanations for your results?
- How do your results compare with those of similar programs?
- Have the different data collection methods used to measure your progress shown similar results?
- Are your results consistent with theories supported by previous research?
- Are your results similar to what you expected? If not, why do you think they may be different?

✓ Checklist for justifying your conclusions

- Analyze data using appropriate techniques.
- Check data for errors.
- Consider issues of context when interpreting data.
- Describe plausible mechanisms or pathways toward change.
- Assess results against available literature.
- Compare different methods for consistent findings.
- Consider alternative explanations.
- Compare evaluation results with those of similar programs.
- Use existing standards (e.g., *Healthy People 2010* objectives) as a starting point for comparisons.
- Compare program outcomes with those of previous years.
- Compare actual with intended outcomes.
- Document potential biases.
- Examine the limitations of the evaluation.

Resources

1. CDC Evaluation Working Group
   www.cdc.gov/eval

6 Ensure Use of Evaluation Findings and Share Lessons Learned

Making recommendations

Once you analyze and interpret your findings, you will need to make some recommendations for action based on those findings. These recommendations will depend on the audience (Box 4). Therefore, it is critical to involve your stakeholders in the early stages of the evaluation so that the recommendations that you eventually make are relevant and useful to them. You need to know the information your stakeholders want and what is important to them. Their feedback early on in the evaluation will make their eventual support of your recommendations more likely.

The purpose of your evaluation (e.g., to improve your program, demonstrate its effectiveness, or demonstrate accountability to stakeholders) will also shape how you frame your recommendations. Here are some examples of recommendations for different audiences:

Potential audiences for recommendations
- Local programs.
- The state health department.
- City councils.
- State legislators.
- Schools.
- Workplace owners.
- Parents.
- Police departments or enforcement agencies.
- Restaurant managers.
- Health care providers.
- Smoking-cessation programs.
- Contractors.
- Health insurance agencies.
- Retailers.
- Youth advocacy groups.

Box 4

Audience: Local counter-marketing program
Purpose of evaluation: Improve program efforts.
Recommendation: Thirty-five percent of African Americans in Region 2 recalled the content of counter-marketing messages. To meet the current objective of a 50% recall rate among this

population group, we recommend developing culturally appropriate media messages and increasing the number of messages targeted to the African American media market in this region.

Audience: Schools/school boards/school administrations.
Purpose of evaluation: Demonstrate effectiveness; improve program efforts.
Recommendation: Although all schools in School District A have implemented CDC-recommended tobacco-free guidelines, only 10% of these schools actively enforce the guidelines. We recommend increasing the number of enforcement activities in School District A. One way to do this is to have the school boards work with local coalitions to provide incentives and commendations for exemplary schools; another is to designate school enforcement officials.

Audience: Legislators.
Purpose of evaluation: Demonstrate effectiveness.
Recommendation: Last year, a targeted education and media campaign about the dangers of ETS and the benefits of smoke-free homes was conducted across the state. Eighty percent of adults were reached by the campaign and reported having smoke-free home rules—a twofold increase from the year before. We recommend the campaign be continued and expanded to include smoke-free automobiles.

Audience: City council.
Purpose of evaluation: Demonstrate effectiveness.
Recommendation: In June of this past year, City C passed a complete ban on smoking in bars and restaurants. Data from our smoke-free-air hotline indicate that 30% of establishments are still not complying with this new ordinance. We recommend that you incorporate compliance checks for this ordinance into the city's health-inspection site visits, apply penalties for violation, and citations for compliance.

Audience: Funding source.
Purpose of evaluation: Demonstrate fiscal accountability.
Recommendation: For the past year, the tobacco control program has worked through local coalitions, educational campaigns, and media efforts to increase awareness and support for smoke-free indoor air policies. As a result, public support for strong smoke-free indoor air policies has increased to 85%,

up from 70% last year, and there has been a 25% increase in the number of workplaces with voluntary smoke-free policies. We recommend continued support for a comprehensive program that includes efforts to address the dangers of ETS and the need for policy change.

Audience: Legislators.
Purpose of evaluation: Monitor trends.
Recommendation: During the past 5 years, smoking-cessation attempts by young adults have decreased. Only 10% of young adult smokers attempted to quit smoking in the past year. We recommend that the program focus on targeting smoking-cessation messages and making cessation services available to young adults across the state.

Sharing the results and the lessons learned from evaluation

After you have decided on the recommendations, the next step is to share the evaluation results with your stakeholders and others who should be aware of the information (Box 4).

Dissemination is the process of communicating either the procedures or the lessons learned from an evaluation in a timely, unbiased, and consistent manner. Planning effective communication requires considering the timing, style, tone, message source, vehicle, and format of information products.

An evaluation report tailored to your audience is an appropriate method for communicating and disseminating the results of the evaluation. The evaluation report must clearly, succinctly, and impartially communicate all parts of the evaluation (Box 5). The report should be written so that it is easy to understand. It need not be lengthy or technical. You should also consider oral presentations tailored to various audiences. Examples of evaluation reports available on the Internet are listed under "Resources" at the end of this chapter.

Tips for writing and disseminating your evaluation report(s)[3]

- Tailor the report to your audience; you may need a different version of your report for each segment of your audience.
- Describe essential features of the program.
- Summarize the stakeholder roles and involvement.
- Explain the focus of the evaluation and its limitations.
- Summarize the evaluation plan and procedures.
- List the strengths and weaknesses of the evaluation.
- Present clear and succinct results and recommendations.
- List the advantages and disadvantages of the recommendations.
- Remove technical jargon.
- Use examples, illustrations, graphics, and stories.
- Verify that the report is unbiased and accurate.
- Provide interim and final reports to intended users in time for use.
- Distribute reports to as many stakeholders as possible.

Box 5

A traditional outline for an evaluation report might look like this:

Executive Summary

Background and Purpose
Program background
Evaluation rationale
Program description

Evaluation Methods
Design
Sampling procedures
Measures or indicators
Data-collection procedures
Data-processing procedures
Analysis
Limitations

Results

Discussion and Recommendations

Appendices

Using the information

The ultimate purpose of program evaluation is to use the information to improve programs. The purpose(s) you identified early in the evaluation process should guide the use of the evaluation results. The evaluation results can be used to demonstrate the effectiveness of your program, identify ways to improve your program, modify program planning, demonstrate accountability, and justify funding.

Additional uses include the following:

- To demonstrate to legislators or other stakeholders that resources are being well spent and that the program is effective.

- To aid in forming budgets and justify the allocation of resources.

- To compare outcomes with those of previous years.

- To compare actual outcomes with intended outcomes.

- To suggest realistic intended outcomes.

- To support annual and long-range planning.

- To focus attention on issues important to your program.

- To promote your program.

- To identify partners for collaborations.

- To enhance the image of your program.

Activities that promote the use of evaluation findings[23]

- Design the evaluation from the start to achieve intended uses by intended users.

- Prepare stakeholders for eventual use by rehearsing how different conclusions could affect program operations.

- Provide continuous feedback to stakeholders about interim findings and decisions to be made that might affect the likelihood of use.

- Schedule follow-up meetings with intended users to facilitate the transfer of evaluation findings into strategic decision making.

6. Ensure Use of Evaluation Findings and Share Lessons Learned

- To retain or increase funding.
- To provide direction for program staff.
- To identify training and technical assistance needs.

Evaluation is a practical tool that states can use to inform programs' efforts and assess their impact. Program evaluation should be well integrated into the day-to-day planning, implementation, and management of public health programs. Program evaluation complements CDC's operating principles for public health, which include using science as a basis for decision making and action, expanding the quest for social equity, performing effectively as a service agency, and making efforts outcome-oriented. These principles highlight the need for programs to develop clear plans, inclusive partnerships, and feedback systems that support ongoing improvement. CDC is committed to providing additional tools and technical assistance to states and tobacco control partners to build and enhance their capacity for evaluation.

> ✓ **Checklist for ensuring that evaluation findings are used and sharing lessons learned**
>
> - Identify strategies to increase the likelihood that evaluation findings will be used.
> - Identify strategies to reduce the likelihood that information will be misinterpreted.
> - Provide continuous feedback to the program.
> - Prepare stakeholders for the eventual use of evaluation findings.
> - Identify training and technical assistance needs.
> - Use evaluation findings to support annual and long-range planning.
> - Use evaluation findings to promote your program.
> - Use evaluation findings to enhance the public image of your program.
> - Schedule follow-up meetings to facilitate the transfer of evaluation conclusions.
> - Disseminate procedures used and lessons learned to stakeholders.
> - Consider interim reports to key audiences.
> - Tailor evaluation reports to audience(s.)
> - Revisit the purpose(s) of the evaluation when preparing recommendations.
> - Present clear and succinct findings in a timely manner.
> - Avoid jargon when preparing or presenting information to stakeholders.
> - Disseminate evaluation findings in several ways.

Resources

1. CDC Evaluation Working Group
   www.cdc.gov/eval

2. Tell Your Story: Guidelines for Preparing an Evaluation Report
   www.dhs.cahwnet.gov/ps/cdic/ccb/TCS/html/
   Evaluation_Resources.htm

3. Criteria for Sound Evaluation Reports
   Online Evaluation Resource Library (OERL)
   www.ctl.sri.com/oerl/reports/reportscrit.html

Sample State Evaluation Reports

- Alaska   www.hss.state.ak.us/dph/tobacco%20report%20final.pdf
- California   www.dhs.ca.gov/tobacco/html/Evaluation_Reports.htm
- Massachusetts   www.state.ma.us/dph/mtcp/report.htm
- Oregon   www.ohd.hr.state.or.us/tobacco/arpt2000/welcome.htm

Sample Youth Tobacco Survey (YTS) Reports

- Arizona   www.tepp.org/evaluation/2000youthsurvey/index.html
- Florida   www.state.fl.us/tobacco (click on research)
- Georgia   www.ph.dhr.state.ga.us
                     www.ph.dhr.state.ga.us/programs/tobacco/pdfs/summaryreport99.pdf
- Iowa   www.idph.state.ia.us/resources.htm
                     www.idph.state.ia.us/sa/Tobacco/iytsfinalreport.pdf
- Kansas   www.kdhe.state.ks.us/tobacco/resources/kyts_99.pdf
- Mississippi   www.msdh.state.ms.us/tobacco
- New Jersey   www.state.nj.us/health/as/smoking.htm
- North Carolina   www.communityhealth.dhhs.state.nc.us/tobacco/Survey/survey.htm
- Oklahoma   www.health.state.ok.us/PROGRAM/tobac/ytsreports.htm
- Tennessee   ftp://170.142.76.180/2000TnYTS.pdf
- Texas   www.tdh.state.tx.us/otpc/stats/statistics.htm
- Wisconsin   www.dhfs.state.wi.us/health/Tobaccocontrol/INDEX.htm

> The resources listed here include links to some nongovernmental organizations' Web sites. These sites are provided solely as examples. Links do not constitute an endorsement of these organizations' materials or programs by CDC or the federal government. CDC is not responsible for the content of any individual organization's Web pages found at these links.

References

1. Centers for Disease Control and Prevention. Smoking-attributable mortality and years of potential life lost—United States, 1984. *MMWR* 1997;46(20):441–51.

2. *Best Practices for Comprehensive Tobacco Control Programs.* Atlanta GA: Centers for Disease Control and Prevention, National Center for Chronic Disease Prevention and Health Promotion, Office on Smoking and Health;1999. Available from: URL: www.cdc.gov/tobacco/bestprac.htm

3. Centers for Disease Control and Prevention. Framework for program evaluation in public health practice. *MMWR* 1999;48(No. RR-11):1–40.

4. U.S. Department of Health and Human Services. *Healthy People 2010:* 2nd ed. *With Understanding and Improving Health and Objectives for Improving Health.* 2 vols. Washington, DC: U.S. Government Printing Office; 2000. Available from: URL: www.health.gov/healthypeople

5. Centers for Disease Control and Prevention. Medical-care expenditures attributable to cigarette smoking—United States, 1993. *MMWR* 1994;43(26):469–72.

6. Herdman R, Hewitt M, Laschover M. *Smoking-Related Deaths and Financial Costs: Office of Technology Assessment Estimates for 1990*—OTA testimony before the Senate Special Committee on Aging. Washington, DC: U.S. Congress, Office of Technology Assessment testimony; May 6, 1993.

7. Centers for Disease Control and Prevention. Cigarette smoking among adults—United States, 1993. *MMWR* 1994;43(50):925–30.

8. *Preventing Tobacco Use Among Young People: A Report of the Surgeon General.* Atlanta, GA: Centers for Disease Control and Prevention, National Center for Chronic Disease Prevention and Health Promotion, Office on Smoking and Health; 1994. [Reprinted, with corrections, July 1994.]

9. Centers for Disease Control and Prevention. Projected smoking-related deaths among youth—United States. *MMWR* 1996;45(44):971–4.

10. Ernster VL, Grady DG, Greene JC, Walsh M, Robertson P, Daniels TE, et al. Smokeless tobacco use and health effects among baseball players. *JAMA* 1990;264(2):218–24.

11. Tomar SL, Winn DM, Swango PA, Giovino GA, Kleinman DV. Oral mucosal smokeless tobacco lesions among adolescents in the United States. *J Dental Res* 1997;76(6):1277–86.

12. National Cancer Institute. Cigars: health effects and trends. In: *Smoking and Tobacco Control Monograph No. 9*. Bethesda, MD: National Institutes of Health, National Cancer Institute; 1998. (NIH Pub. No. 98-4302)

13. Centers for Disease Control and Prevention. Youth tobacco surveillance—United States, 1998–1999. *MMWR* 2000;49(SS-10):1–93.

14. Davis RM. Exposure to environmental tobacco smoke: identifying and protecting those at risk. *JAMA* 1998;280(22):1947–9.

15. National Cancer Institute. Health effects of exposure to environmental tobacco smoke: the report of the California Environmental Protection Agency. In: *Smoking and Tobacco Control Monograph No. 10*. Bethesda, MD: National Institutes of Health, National Cancer Institute; 1999. (NIH Pub. No. 99-4645)

16. Environmental Protection Agency. *Respiratory Health Effects of Passive Smoking: Lung Cancer and Other Disorders*. Washington, DC: Environmental Protection Agency, Office of Research and Development, Office of Air and Radiation; 1992. (Pub. No. EPA/600/6-90/006F)

17. Green LW, Eriksen MP, Bailey L, Husten C. Achieving the implausible in the next decade's tobacco control objectives. *Am J Public Health* 2000;90(3):337–9.

18. Patton MQ. *Utilization-Focused Evaluation: The New Century Text*. 3rd ed. Thousand Oaks, CA: Sage Publications; 1997.

19. WHO European Working Group on Health Promotion Evaluation. *Health Promotion Evaluation: Recommendations to Policy-Makers: Report of the WHO European Working Group on Health Promotion Evaluation*. Copenhagen, Denmark: World Health Organization, Regional Office for Europe; 1998. Available from: URL: www.who.dk/document/e60706.pdf.

20. Joint Committee on Standards for Educational Evaluation. *The Program Evaluation Standards: How to Assess Evaluations of Educational Programs*. 2nd ed. Thousand Oaks, CA: Sage Publications; 1994.

21. Centers for Disease Control and Prevention. *Prevention Research Centers: At a Glance 2001.* Available from: URL: www.cdc.gov/prc/glance.htm.

22. Green LW, George MA, Daniel M, Frankish CJ, Herbert CP, Bowie WR, et al. *Study of Participatory Research in Health Promotion: Review and Recommendations for the Development of Participatory Research in Health Promotion in Canada.* Ottawa, Canada: Royal Society of Canada; 1995.

23. The University of Texas–Houston Health Sciences Center School of Public Health and The Texas Health Department. *Practical Evaluation of Public Health Programs.* Atlanta, GA: Centers for Disease Control and Prevention. Available from: URL: www.cdc.gov/phtn/Pract-Eval/workbook.htm.

24. Green LW, Kreuter MW. *Health Promotion Planning: An Educational and Ecological Approach.* 3rd ed. Mountain View, CA: Mayfield Publishing Company; 1999.

25. Green LW, Ottoson JM. *Community and Population Health.* 8th ed. Boston, MA: WCB/McGraw-Hill; 1999.

26. Green LW, Lewis FM. *Measurement and Evaluation in Health Education and Health Promotion.* Palo Alto, CA: Mayfield Publishing Company; 1986.

27. *Measuring Program Outcomes: A Practical Approach.* Alexandria, VA: United Way of America; 1996.

28. Bond SL, Boyd SE, Rapp KA. *Taking Stock: A Practical Guide to Evaluating Your Own Programs.* Chapel Hill, NC: Horizon Research; 1997.

29. The Health Communication Unit at the Centre for Health Promotion, University of Toronto. *Evaluating Health Promotion Programs.* Toronto, Ontario, Canada: The Banting Institute; 1998. Available from: URL: www.thcu.ca/infoandresources/publications/Eval%20HPP-020801.pdf.

Glossary

Accountability: The responsibility of program managers and staff to provide evidence to stakeholders and funding agencies that a program is effective and in conformance with its coverage, service, legal, and fiscal requirements.

Accuracy: The extent to which an evaluation is truthful or valid in what it says about a program, project, or material.

Activities: The actual events or actions that take place as a part of the program.

Attitudes: People's biases, inclinations, or tendencies that influence their response to situations, activities, people, or program goals.

Baseline information: Data gathered on the target population before a tobacco control program begins.

Capacity: The resources (e.g., competent staff, appropriate data-collection systems, sufficient funding) to conduct an evaluation.

Case study: An intensive, detailed description and analysis of a single project or program in the context of its environment.

Competency: The knowledge and experience needed to conduct surveillance and evaluation.

Cross-sectional data: Observations collected at one point in time.

Data: Documented information or evidence of any kind.

Data analysis: The process of systematically applying statistical and logical techniques to describe, summarize, and compare data.

Data-collection instrument: A form or set of forms used to collect information for an evaluation (e.g., questionnaires, interview guides, intake forms, participation logs, attendance records). It may be developed specifically for an evaluation or modified from existing instruments.

Data-collection plan: A written document describing the specific procedures to be used to gather the evaluation data. The document describes who collects the information, when and where it is collected, and how it is obtained.

Database: A collection of information that has been systematically organized for easy access and analysis. Databases typically are computerized.

Dissemination: The process of communicating either the procedures or the lessons learned from an evaluation in a timely, unbiased, and consistent manner.

Executive summary: A nontechnical summary statement designed to provide a quick overview of the full-length report on which it is based.

Experimental designs: In evaluation, methods that involve randomly assigning people in the target population to one of two or more groups in order to eliminate the effects of history and maturation. The program's effects are measured by comparing the change in one group or set of groups with the change in another group or set of groups.

Evaluation plan: A written document describing the overall approach or design that will be used to guide an evaluation. It includes what will be done, how it will be done, who will do it, when it will done, why the evaluation is being conducted, and how the findings will likely be used.

Feasibility: The extent to which resources allow an evaluation to be conducted.

Focus group: A group of people selected for their relevance to an evaluation that is engaged by a trained facilitator in a series of discussions designed for sharing insights, ideas, and observations on a topic of concern.

Indicator: A specific, observable, and measurable characteristic or change that shows the progress a program is making toward achieving a specified outcome.

Infrastructure: All the components necessary to conduct an evaluation (e.g., experienced staff, adequate funding).

Inputs: Resources that go into a program.

Logic model: A systematic and visual way to present the perceived relationships among the resources you have to operate the program, the activities you plan to do, and the changes or results you hope to achieve.

Longitudinal data: Observations collected over a period of time; the sample (instances or cases) may or may not be the same each time but the population remains constant.

Objectives: Statements describing the results to be achieved and the manner in which these results will be achieved.

Outputs: The direct products of program activities; immediate measures of what the program did.

Outcomes: The results of program operations or activities; the effects triggered by the program. (For example, increased knowledge, changed attitudes or beliefs, reduced tobacco use, reduced tobacco-related morbidity and mortality.)

Outcome evaluation: the systematic collection of information to assess the impact of a program, present conclusions about the merit or worth of a program, and make recommendations about future program direction or improvement.

Posttest: A test or measurement taken after services or activities have ended. It is compared with the results of a pretest to show evidence of the effects or changes resulting from the services or activities being evaluated.

Pretest: A test or measurement taken before services or activities begin. It is compared with the results of a posttest to show evidence of the effects of the services or activities being evaluated. A pretest can be used to obtain baseline data.

Process evaluation: The systematic collection of information to document and assess how a program was implemented and operates.

Program evaluation: The systematic collection of information about the activities, characteristics, and outcomes of programs to make judgments about the program, improve program effectiveness, and/or inform decisions about future program development.

Program goal: A statement of the overall mission or purpose(s) of the program.

Propriety: The extent to which the evaluation has been conducted in a manner that evidences uncompromising adherence to the highest principles and ideals (including professional ethics, civil law, moral code, and contractual agreements).

Qualitative methods: Ways of collecting information on the knowledge, attitudes, beliefs, and behaviors of the target population. In general, information gathered using qualitative methods is not given a numerical value.

Quasi-experimental design: In evaluation, methods that do not involve randomly assigning members of the target population either to an intervention or to a comparison group.

Resources: Assets available and anticipated for operations. They include people, equipment, facilities, and other things used to plan, implement, and evaluate public programs whether or not paid for directly by public funds.

Sample: A subset of people in a particular population.

Sampling frame: Complete list of all people or households in the target population.

Stakeholder: People or organizations who are invested in the program or who are interested in the results of the evaluation or what will be done with results of the evaluation.

Standard: A principle commonly agreed to by experts in the conduct and use of an evaluation for the measure of the value or quality of an evaluation (e.g. accuracy, feasibility, propriety, utility).

Surveillance: The ongoing, systematic collection, analysis, and interpretation of data (e.g., regarding agent/hazard, risk factor, exposure, health event) essential to the planning, implementation, and evaluation of public health practice, closely integrated with the timely dissemination of these data to those responsible for prevention and control.

Glossary

Survey: A quantitative (nonexperimental) method of collecting information on the target population at one point in time. Surveys may be conducted by interview (in person or by telephone) or by questionnaire.

Utility: The extent to which an evaluation produces and disseminates reports that inform relevant audiences and have beneficial impact on their work.

Appendix A

Surveillance and Evaluation Data Resources for Comprehensive Tobacco Control Programs

Appendix A

Surveillance and Evaluation Data Resources for Comprehensive Tobacco Control Programs

Appendix A is an at-a-glance compilation of sources of data useful for tobacco control programs that are conducting surveillance or evaluation. Our objective is to provide basic information on each data source to assist state tobacco control programs in identifying data that are relevant to planning, monitoring, and evaluation. The data sources listed here provide a wide variety of tobacco-related information. For example, the NTCP Chronicle and local program monitoring have useful data on programmatic activities; restaurant and work-site surveys, key informant surveys, and third-party payer surveys have data on environmental policies and indicators; the Youth Tobacco Survey, Adult Tobacco Survey, and media evaluation surveys have data on individual knowledge, attitudes, and behaviors; and the cancer registries and hospital discharge records have data on health outcomes.

Data sources checked as "used frequently and comparable across states" are often used to help states develop tobacco program objectives. Data from these sources can be used to compare program impact and outcomes with those of other states and the nation as a whole.

The data sources are organized under major categories: national and state surveys, registries and vital statistics, and topic-specific tools. The columns in each table provide the following information:

Column 1: Data Source

- Name of the data source.

- General description of the data source.

Column 2: Tobacco-Related Indicators

- Topics on which information is available. For example, environmental tobacco smoke, tobacco-related policies, brand preferences, type of tobacco product (cigarette, cigar, pipe, smokeless tobacco, or bidi).

- The range in the number of tobacco-related questions included in the survey instrument, or—if applicable—within the core instrument, modules, or supplements.

Column 3: Sampling Frame

- The level of information available: national, state, community, or local.

- Details on target or study population (e.g., adults, pregnant women) or factors that were studied (e.g., media campaigns, number of telephone calls, hospital records).

Column 4: Methodology (a); Frequency (b); Years Completed (c)

- (a) Study design and data collection mode (e.g., random sample, telephone survey; convenience sample, unannounced interviews).

- (b) How often surveys are conducted (e.g., annually, periodically).

- (c) The years when data were collected.

Column 5: Comments

- Additional useful information.

Column 6: Contact

- Phone number or Internet address of the organization where you can obtain more information.

Not all of the data sources are available in every state. Consequently, some states may consider investing funds to develop systems to address gaps in data. New data-collection systems should be directly relevant to state programmatic goals, objectives, and activities. However, prior to choosing data sources or investing resources to develop new data systems, programs should consider some of the following issues: timeliness, frequency, comparability, credibility, and available resources. For more information on these considerations, please see CDC's 2001 publication *An Introduction to Evaluation: Planning, Implementation and Use*, or contact the CDC's Office on Smoking and Health's State Surveillance and Evaluation Team (telephone: 770-488-5703).

Appendix A

Table 1. National and State Surveys and Tools

Data Source	Tobacco-Related Indicators	Sampling Frame	Methodology (a), Frequency (b), Years Completed (c)	Comments	Contact
✓ **Adult Tobacco Survey (ATS)** ■ Provides data on adult tobacco use, knowledge, attitudes, and tobacco use prevention and control policies. ■ Individual state ATSs have been conducted in 15 states since 1986.	*Topics*: ■ Cigarette, cigar, pipe, bidi, kretek, and smokeless tobacco use. ■ ETS exposure and policies. ■ Cessation behaviors. ■ Health and social influences, parental involvement, media exposure, and other policy issues. *Number of questions*: From 64 to 168.	State level. *Subjects*: Adults aged 18 or older.	a) Random design, telephone survey. b) Periodic.	State tobacco programs should work with BRFSS coordinators to design and implement an ATS. Centers for Disease Control and Prevention (CDC), Office on Smoking and Health, has developed a standardized instrument and optional questions for state use.	Office on Smoking and Health, Centers for Disease Control and Prevention. (770) 488-5703. State health departments.
Adult Use of Tobacco Survey (AUTS) ■ Provides descriptive information on knowledge, attitudes, and behaviors related to tobacco use prevention and control.	*Topics*: ■ Cigarette, cigar, pipe, smokeless tobacco use. ■ Age of initiation. ■ Exposure to ETS. ■ Brand preference. ■ Cessation behavior. ■ Knowledge and attitudes.	National level. *Subjects*: Adults aged 18 or older.	a) Random design, telephone survey. b) Periodic. c) 1964, 1966, 1970, 1986.	Most recent survey was completed in 1986.	National Technical Information Service. (703) 605-6585. www.ntis.gov Office on Smoking and Health, Centers for Disease Control and Prevention. (770) 488-5703. www.cdc.gov/tobacco
✓ **Behavioral Risk Factor Surveillance System (BRFSS)** ■ Provides descriptive data on health risk behaviors, including tobacco use and preventive health measures in general. ■ The survey began in 1984 with 15 states participating. Since 1996, all 50 states have participated.	*Topics*: The tobacco topics vary by year. In 2001, they were— ■ Cigarette, cigar, smokeless tobacco, pipe, and bidi use. ■ Age of initiation. ■ Cessation behaviors. ■ ETS policies and rules. *Number of questions*: From 5 to 17.	State level. *Subjects*: Adults age 18 or older.	a) Random design, telephone survey. b) Annual. c) 1984–present.	1996: CDC changed its definition of a *cigarette smoker*. 1998: tobacco topics added to the optional modules, in addition to those in the core questionnaire. State tobacco programs should work with BRFSS coordinators to have tobacco-related questions added to state survey.	Division of Adult and Community Health, Centers for Disease Control and Prevention. (770) 488-2455. www.cdc.gov/nccdphp/BRFSS State health departments.

Table 1
✓ Data are frequently used and comparable across states.
Abbreviations: ETS = environmental tobacco smoke.

Table 1. National and State Surveys and Tools

Data Source	Tobacco-Related Indicators	Sampling Frame	Methodology (a), Frequency (b), Years Completed (c)	Comments	Contact
Cancer Prevention Study (CPSII) ■ Provides data on age and cause of death for a prospective cohort of 1.2 million people nationwide since 1982. ■ Information about tobacco use, medical history, dietary habits, environment, and other health determinants are recorded and related to causes of death.	*Topics:* ■ Cigarette use. ■ Age of initiation. ■ Brand preference. ■ Degree of inhalation. *Number of questions:* From 3 to 9.	National level. *Subjects:* Adults aged 35 or older.	a) Cohort study with convenience sample, self-administered survey. b) Biennial follow-up. c) September 1982–present.	More representative of middle class, white Americans (96% of sample) than the national population as a whole.	American Cancer Society. (404) 329-7762. www.cancer.org
✓ **Current Population Survey (CPS)** ■ Provides a comprehensive body of data on the employment and unemployment experience of the U.S. population, classified by age, sex, race, and a variety of other characteristics. ■ Periodic supplements have included tobacco-related measures.	*Topics:* Periodic measures have included— ■ Cigarette, pipe, cigar, and smokeless use. ■ Age of initiation. ■ ETS exposure. ■ Cessation behavior. *Number of questions:* From 5 to 46.	National and state levels. *Subjects:* People aged 15 or older.	a) Random design, household interview with telephone follow-up. b) Periodic. c) 1968–present.	Includes self-reported and proxy-reported data, data from Tobacco Use Supplement available 1992–1993, 1995–1996, and 1998–1999.	National Cancer Institute. (301) 435-3848. http://appliedresearch.cancer.gov/RiskFactor/tobacco/index.html U.S. Census Bureau. (301) 457-4100 www.census.gov/apsd/techdoc/cps/cps-main.html

Table 1 (continued)

✓Data are frequently used and comparable across states.
Abbreviations: ETS = environmental tobacco smoke.

Appendix A

Table 1. National and State Surveys and Tools

Data Source	Tobacco-Related Indicators	Sampling Frame	Methodology (a), Frequency (b), Years Completed (c)	Comments	Contact
Monitoring the Future (MTF) ■ Provides annual data on behaviors, knowledge, attitudes, and values related to the use of an array of psychoactive substances, both illicit and licit, among American secondary school students, college students, and young adults.	*Topics:* ■ Cigarette use. ■ Age of initiation. ■ Cessation behavior. ■ Brand preference. ■ Youth access. ■ Enforcement. ■ Media awareness. *Number of questions:* From 3 to 64.	National level. *Subjects:* 8th, 10th, and 12th grade students, and young adults.	a) Random design, self-administered school-based survey, follow-up survey mailed to cohort population. b) Annual. c) 1975–present.	12th graders surveyed since 1975, and 8th and 10th graders surveyed since 1991. Annual follow-up questionnaires are mailed to a nationally representative sample of each high school graduating class for a number of years after their initial participation. Prevalence and trend data available for cohort population that is now between 35–40 years old.	National Institute on Drug Abuse. (888) 741-7242. www.monitoringthefuture.org www.isr.umich.edu
National Health and Nutrition Examination Survey (NHANES) ■ Provides data on the health and diet of the U.S. population nationwide. Includes information on the prevalence of selected diseases and risk factors; the population's awareness, knowledge, and attitudes; and prevention and control of selected diseases. The survey also includes a medical examination for participants and a laboratory component.	*Topics:* ■ Cigarette, cigar, pipe, smokeless tobacco use. ■ ETS exposure. ■ Cessation behavior. ■ Brand preference. ■ Serum continue measurements. *Number of questions:* From 35 to 62.	National level. *Subjects:* Households, families, and individuals aged 4 or older.	a) Random design; household and mobile unit survey. (b and c) Periodic: ■ 1971–1975 (NHANES I) ■ 1976–1980 (NHANES II) ■ 1988–1994 (NHANES III) Annual: ■ 1999–present.	This is the only major survey that provides serum cotinine measurements (for subjects age 4 and older). Low income persons, adolescents 12–19 years, persons 60+ years of age, African Americans and Mexican Americans are oversampled to provide significant data for these groups.	National Center for Health Statistics, Centers for Disease Control and Prevention. (301) 458-4681. www.cdc.gov/NCHS/nhanes

Table 1 (continued)
Abbreviations: ETS = environmental tobacco smoke.

Introduction to Program Evaluation for Comprehensive Tobacco Control Programs

Table 1. National and State Surveys and Tools

Data Source	Tobacco-Related Indicators	Sampling Frame	Methodology (a), Frequency (b), Years Completed (c)	Comments	Contact
✓ **National Health Interview Survey (NHIS)** • Provides data on U.S. health issues, including incidence and prevalence of acute and chronic conditions and people's knowledge and attitudes about health status and health care use. This is the primary source of data on current health issues in the United States. In additional to the basic survey protocol, each year there are supplements to the survey to collect information on specific topics.	*Topics:* • Cigarette, cigar, pipe, bidi, smokeless tobacco use. • Age of initiation. • Cessation behavior. • ETS policies. • Exposure. *Number of questions:* From 18 to 55.	National level. *Subjects:* Adults aged 18 or older. In 1997, questionnaire redesign was fully implemented.	a) Random design, household survey. (b and c) Periodic: • 1965–1987. Annual. • 1990–present.	Tobacco measures are located in core questionnaire and optional modules. 1997 redesign tripled state-specific sample size. Hispanics and African Americans are oversampled. Data from NHIS is used to monitor progress in achieving national *Healthy People 2010* tobacco objectives related to adults.	National Center for Health Statistics, Centers for Disease Control and Prevention. (301) 458-4001. www.cdc.gov/nchs/data
National Household Survey on Drug Abuse (NHSDA) • Provides data on the prevalence, patterns, knowledge and attitudes, and consequences of drug and alcohol use and abuse in the U.S. (including tobacco).	*Topics:* • Cigarette, cigar, pipe, and smokeless tobacco use. • Age of initiation. *Number of questions:* From 6 to 12.	National level. *Subjects:* People aged 12 or older (12–17, 18–35, ≥36). In 1998, direct state-level estimates were produced for 8 states, and indirect estimates were produced for others.	a) Random design, household survey. (b and c) Periodic: • 1971–1988. Annual. • 1990–present.	The survey provides estimates of the rate and number of tobacco users by gender, race/ethnicity, and region. State estimates are available for prevalence of tobacco use only.	Substance Abuse and Mental Health Services Administration. (301) 443-6239. www.samhsa.gov/statistics

Table 1 (continued)

✓Data are frequently used and comparable across states.

Abbreviations: ATS = Adult Tobacco Survey. BRFSS = Behavioral Risk Factor Surveillance System. ETS = environmental tobacco smoke.

Table 1. National and State Surveys and Tools

Data Source	Tobacco-Related Indicators	Sampling Frame	Methodology (a), Frequency (b), Years Completed (c)	Comments	Contact
National Youth Tobacco Survey (NYTS) ■ Provides data on knowledge, attitudes, and behaviors related to tobacco use.	*Topics:* ■ Cigarette, cigar, pipe, bidi, kretek, smokeless tobacco use. ■ ETS exposure. ■ Media awareness. ■ Cessation behavior. ■ Youth access. *Number of questions:* From 57 to 76.	National level. *Subjects:* Students in grades 6–12.	a) Random design, self-administered in classroom. b) Annual. c) 1999–present.	Includes students in public and private schools. Serves as a national comparison to state YTS results.	American Legacy Foundation. (202) 454-5555. www.americanlegacy.org
National Tobacco Control Program (NTCP) Chronicle ■ Provides data on the tobacco control and prevention activities of all 50 states and the District of Columbia funded through the CDC's NTCP. ■ Information is captured in four key goal areas and selected infrastructure components, including staffing, collaboration, funding, technical assistance and training, and surveillance and evaluation.	*Topics:* Using both quantitative and qualitative indicators, program progress is measured for the key goal areas— ■ Preventing initiation and promoting quitting among youth. ■ Promoting quitting among adults. ■ Eliminating exposure to ETS. ■ Identifying and eliminating disparities.	State level. *Subjects:* Tobacco control programs in 50 states and the District of Columbia.	a) Census, Web-based program monitoring system. b) Completed twice yearly, reporting on previous 6 months of activity. c) Fiscal Year 1999–present.	The NTCP Chronicle collects information on comprehensive tobacco control activities.	Office on Smoking and Health, Centers for Disease Control and Prevention. (770) 488-5703. State health departments.

Table 1 (continued)
Abbreviations: ETS = environmental tobacco smoke. YTS = Youth Tobacco Survey.

Table 1. National and State Surveys and Tools

Data Source	Tobacco-Related Indicators	Sampling Frame	Methodology (a), Frequency (b), Years Completed (c)	Comments	Contact
✓ **Pregnancy Risk Assessment Monitoring System (PRAMS)** ■ Provides ongoing population-based surveillance of selected maternal behaviors, including tobacco use. ■ In 1987, 13 states and the District of Columbia completed the survey. ■ In 2000, 24 states and New York City conducted the survey.	**Topics:** ■ Cigarette use before and during pregnancy and in the child's early infancy. ■ ETS exposure. ■ Cessation counseling **Number of questions:** From 6 to 9.	State level. **Subjects:** Mothers of infants 2–4 months old.	a) Random design, mail survey with telephone follow-up. b) Annual. c) 1988–present.	This is an ongoing survey. Availability of data depends on when states began participating.	Division of Reproductive Health, Centers for Disease Control and Prevention. (770) 488-5227. www.cdc.gov/nccdphp/drh State health departments.
✓ **School Health Education Profiles (SHEP)** ■ Provides information on health education policies and programs through a survey for the lead health educator and a separate survey for the school principal. ■ Formerly a School Tobacco Survey (STS) module for lead health educators and school principals was used to assess tobacco policies and programs. ■ In 2001 the tobacco module was combined with the core surveys for lead health educators and school principals.	**Topics:** The core survey includes all the tobacco questions— (6 questions on the lead health educator questionnaire and 13 questions on the principal questionnaire). ■ School tobacco use policies for students, staff, and visitors. ■ Enforcement of policies. ■ Tobacco prevention curriculum. ■ Parental involvement in tobacco use prevention. ■ Cessation programs. ■ Retailer practices. ■ Tobacco advertising. Different indicators are measured on different versions of the questionnaire. **Number of questions:** From 3 to 39.	State level. **Subjects:** Middle/junior and senior high schools.	a) Random design, mail survey sent to school principals and lead health educators. b) Biennial (even years). c) 1994–present.		Division of Adolescent and School Health, Centers for Disease Control and Prevention. (888) 231-6405. www.cdc.gov/nccdphp/dash Office on Smoking and Health, Centers for Disease Control and Prevention. (770) 488-5703. www.cdc.gov/tobacco

Table 1 (continued)

✓Data are frequently used and comparable across states.
Abbreviations: ETS = environmental tobacco smoke.

Table 1. National and State Surveys and Tools

Data Source	Tobacco-Related Indicators	Sampling Frame	Methodology (a), Frequency (b), Years Completed (c)	Comments	Contact
School Health Policies and Programs Study (SHPPS) ■ Monitors characteristics of health education and school health programs in middle/junior high and senior high schools. ■ These school-based surveys are conducted biennially by state and local education and health agencies using representative samples of elementary, middle/junior high and senior high schools in their jurisdictions.	*Topics:* ■ School tobacco policies. ■ Educational programs and curriculum. ■ Health services. *Number of questions:* From 3 to 35.	State, district, school, classroom levels. *Subjects:* Elementary, middle/junior high, and high schools. State-level information provided by this survey includes only state education policies. Sample size: 1,500 middle schools/ 1,500 high schools.	a) Random sample of school districts, schools, and classrooms of public and private schools grades K-12 using mail surveys at district level and on-site structured interviews at school and classroom level. b) Periodic. c) 1994 and 2000.		Division of Adolescent and School Health, Centers for Disease Control and Prevention. (888) 231-6405. www.cdc.gov/nccdphp/dash/SHPPS
✓ **Smoking Attributable Morbidity, Mortality, & Economic Costs (SAMMEC), software version 3.0** ■ The SAMMEC software programs are Internet-based products designed to calculate the health and economic burden of smoking for adults and infants. ■ The two types of software, Adult SAMMEC and Maternal and Child Health SAMMEC, employ the latest scientific evidence on smoking-related diseases, risks associated with current and former smoking, and the economic costs of smoking.	*Topics:* ■ Calculates smoking-attributable mortality (SAM), years of potential life lost (YPLLs), direct medical expenditures and indirect productivity costs from cigarette smoking among adults. ■ The MCH SAMMEC software calculates SAMs and YPLLs from low birth weight and Sudden Infant Death Syndrome (SIDS), and neonatal medical expenditures.	National and state levels. *Subjects:* Adults aged 35 or older (Adult SAMMEC) and infants aged 1 year or younger (MCH SAMMEC).	a) Current Population Survey data are used to calculate YPLLs and productivity costs associated with SAM. ■ Direct medical care expenditures are estimated using National Medical Expenditure Survey data. ■ Maternal smoking data from PRAMS is used to calculate perinatal SAMs and YPLLs. ■ Health care utilization data from PRAMS and medical claims data are used to calculate smoking-attributable neonatal medical expenditures. c) CDC provides estimates of average annual smoking-attributable mortality and years of potential life lost from 1995-1999 for the nation and 1999 data for states. Direct medical expenditures and mortality-related productivity loss estimates are provided for the nation and states for 1999.	SAMMEC requires a population of at least 400,000 to create statistically valid estimates, and is therefore not useful for producing local-level estimates or estimates of population subgroups (e.g., by race/ethnicity). Internet version will be available by late November 2001.	Office on Smoking and Health, Centers for Disease Control and Prevention. (770) 488-5703. www.cdc.gov/tobacco Division of Reproductive Health, Centers for Disease Control and Prevention. (770) 488-5372. www.cdc.gov/nccdphp/drh

Table 1 (continued)

✓ Data are frequently used and comparable across states.

Abbreviations: MCH = Maternal and Child Health. PRAMS = Pregnancy Risk Assessment Monitoring System.

Table 1. National and State Surveys and Tools

Data Source	Tobacco-Related Indicators	Sampling Frame	Methodology (a), Frequency (b), Years Completed (c)	Comments	Contact
✓ **State Tobacco Activities Tracking & Evaluation (STATE) System** ■ The STATE System is a data warehouse that provides comparable measures on tobacco-use prevention and control from many different types of data sources, including legislative tracking, agricultural and manufacturing, and health consequences and costs. ■ The system allows users to view comprehensive summary information on tobacco use in all 50 states and the District of Columbia.	*Topics:* ■ Adult and youth cigarette, cigar, pipe, and smokeless tobacco use. ■ ETS laws and policies. ■ Youth access laws. ■ Excise taxes. ■ Smoking-attributable costs.	State level.	a) Varies according to data source. c) Prevalence data from mid-1980 until 1999. Smoking attributable cost in 1993 only. Youth access laws and environmental laws from 1996 until 2000. Dates for excise taxes depend on year of enactment in the state.	Provides comprehensive legislative and behavioral data.	Office on Smoking and Health, Centers for Disease Control and Prevention. (770) 488-5703. www.cdc.gov/tobacco
Teenage Attitudes and Practices Survey (TAPS) ■ Provides data on knowledge and attitudes such as perceived benefits and risks of tobacco use among teens.	*Topics:* ■ Cigarette and smokeless tobacco use. ■ Brand preference. ■ Age of initiation. ■ Cessation behavior. ■ Media awareness.	National level. *Subjects:* Youth aged 12–18. 1993 study includes youth aged 10–22.	a) Random design, household survey. b) Periodic. c) 1989 and 1993.	Limitations for this survey include a non-response bias for those re-interviewed in the second survey (those who were re-interviewed were less likely to have been smokers in 1989 than those who could not be re-interviewed). Also, the small number of African American and Hispanic adolescents in the second survey reduces the reliability of the brand preference estimates for those groups. The second survey (1993) included 87% of the respondents from the first survey, as well as youth from a new probability sample.	National Technical Information Service. (703) 605-6585. www.ntis.gov

Table 1 (continued)

✓ Data are frequently used and comparable across states.
Abbreviations: ETS = environmental tobacco smoke.

Appendix A

Table 1. National and State Surveys and Tools

Data Source	Tobacco-Related Indicators	Sampling Frame	Methodology (a), Frequency (b), Years Completed (c)	Comments	Contact
✓ **Youth Risk Behavior Surveillance System (YRBSS)** ■ Provides data on priority health risk behaviors that contribute to leading causes of mortality, morbidity, and social problems among youth and adults in the U.S. ■ The survey monitors six categories of behaviors: 1) tobacco use, 2) alcohol and other drug use, 3) sexual behaviors that contribute to unintended pregnancy and sexually transmitted disease, 4) dietary behaviors, 5) physical activity, and 6) behaviors that result in violence and unintentional injuries.	**Topics:** ■ Cigarette, cigar, and smokeless tobacco use. ■ Age of initiation. ■ Youth access. ■ Enforcement. ■ Cessation behavior. **Number of questions:** 12.	National, state, and large city levels. **Subjects:** Students in grades 9–12.	a) Random design, self-administered in classroom. (b and c) 1990. Biennial (odd years). 1991–present.	Data from YRBSS is used to monitor progress in achieving national *Healthy People 2010* tobacco objectives related to young people.	Division of Adolescent and School Health. Centers for Disease Control and Prevention. (888) 231-6405. www.cdc.gov/yrbs
✓ **Youth Tobacco Survey (YTS)** ■ Provides data on youth knowledge, attitudes and behaviors, and major tobacco indicators. In 1998, the survey was administered in 3 states, 13 states in 1999, 29 states in 2000, and over 20 states are expected to administer the survey in 2001.	**Topics:** ■ Cigarette, cigar, pipe, and smokeless tobacco use. ■ Age of initiation ■ Media awareness. ■ Youth access. ■ Cessation behavior. ■ ETS exposure. ■ School curriculum. **Number of questions:** 63.	State level. **Subjects:** Students in grades 6–8 and 9–12.	a) Random design, self-administered in classroom. b) Conducted based on states' programmatic needs and in coordination with their surveillance and evaluation plans.	Schools selected with probability proportional to size, classrooms chosen randomly. Some states conduct the survey in middle schools or high schools only, some in both. It is recommended that states include state-added questions to the core questionnaire.	Office on Smoking and Health. Centers for Disease Control and Prevention. (770) 488-5703. www.cdc.gov/tobacco

Table 1 (continued)
✓Data are frequently used and comparable across states.
Abbreviations: ETS = environmental tobacco smoke.

Table 2. Registries and Vital Statistics

Data Source	Tobacco-Related Indicators	Sampling Frame	Methodology (a), Frequency (b), Years Completed (c)	Comments	Contact
Birth Certificate Data<ul><li>Provides data on tobacco use by pregnant women.</li></ul>	*Topics:*<ul><li>Indicators vary by state.</li><li>Smoking during pregnancy.</li></ul>	State level. *Subjects:* Women who recently gave birth.	a) Varies by state. Certificates completed by physicians, registered nurse, or patient at hospitals and clinics. Information may be obtained in person or based on patient's chart. b) Varies by state. c) Data is available since 1989 for some states.	Tobacco use may be under-reported. May be used at the sub-state level (i.e., counties, health districts).	State health departments.
Cancer Registry Data<ul><li>Provides incidence data on smoking-related cancers.</li><li>Comprehensive, timely, and accurate data about cancer incidence, stage at diagnosis, first course of treatment, and deaths.</li></ul>	*Topics:* Indicators vary by state, since there are no national standards on reporting tobacco use history.<ul><li>Smoking status.</li><li>Use of other tobacco products.</li></ul>	State level. *Subjects:* Adults and children.	a) Passive surveillance system from hospitals, physicians' offices, therapeutic radiation facilities, freestanding surgical centers, and pathology laboratories. Data are collected in person. b) Varies by state.	The registry systems vary across states. There is potential for under-reporting since physicians complete the forms and may not have access to patients' full medical records.	North American Association of Central Cancer Registries. www.naaccr.org Cancer Prevention and Control. Centers for Disease Control and Prevention. (888) 842-6355. www.cdc.gov/CANCER/npcr
Death Certificate Data<ul><li>Provides data on causes of death.</li><li>Used to assess tobacco-related mortality.</li></ul>	*Topics:* Data on tobacco use varies by state.<ul><li>ICD codes.</li><li>Tobacco-use status.</li></ul>	State level. *Subjects:* Deceased adults and children.	a) Certificates completed by physicians at hospitals and clinics. Demographics provided by the funeral director. b) Federal efforts to standardize reporting began in 1946 in the Bureau of the Census and moved to the National Center for Health Statistics in 1950.	Possible under-reporting of tobacco use because of physician bias. May be used at the sub-state level (i.e., counties, health districts) or in SAMMEC for estimates of state impact.	National Center for Health Statistics, Cancer Prevention and Control. Centers for Disease Control and Prevention. (301) 458-4681. www.cdc.gov/nchs

Table 2
Abbreviations: ICD = International Classification of Disease. SAMMEC = Smoking Attributable Morbidity, Mortality, and Economic Costs.

Appendix A

Table 3. Topic-Specific Tools: Health Systems and Clinical Settings

Data Source	Tobacco-Related Indicators	Sampling Frame	Methodology (a), Frequency (b), Years Completed (c)	Comments	Contact
Health Provider Surveys ■ Monitors medical practices and policies.	*Topics:* ■ Cessation policies. ■ Clinical practices related to tobacco use.	*Subjects:* Physicians, nurses, physician assistants, dentists.	a) Varies. b) Varies.		State health departments. State licensing bureau. State managed care association.
Health Plan Employer Data and Information Set (HEDIS) ■ Provides a set of standardized performance measures designed to give purchasers and consumers the information they need to compare the performance of managed health care plans. ■ Health care providers who advise smokers to quit smoking is the performance measure of interest.	*Topics:* ■ Cigarette use. ■ Cessation counseling.	National level. *Subjects:* Commercial health plan members, Medicaid and Medicare recipients.	a) Random design. Mail survey. c) 1996–1999.	Small sample size, low response rate, response bias, and recall bias. 1999 is the most recent data set. Archived data sets may be available for purchase.	National Committee for Quality Assurance. (888) 275-7585. www.ncqa.org
Hospital Discharge Data ■ Provides background information on patient and morbidity through discharge diagnoses, number of days of hospitalization, and treatment.	*Topics:* ■ Health effects. ■ Length of stay.	Hospital records.	a) Varies. b) Continuous.	Information on smoking status is usually not available or may be misclassified.	State health departments.

Table 3

Table 3. Topic-Specific Tools: Health Systems and Clinical Settings

Data Source	Tobacco-Related Indicators	Sampling Frame	Methodology (a), Frequency (b), Years Completed (c)	Comments	Contact
MarketScan Database ■ Provides health data on private companies' insured employees and their dependents, early retirees, ex-employees still on COBRA, and Medicare-eligible retirees with employer-provided Medicare Supplemental plans.	*Topics:* ■ Paid claims and encounter data related to cessation services.	National level. *Subjects:* Employees and dependents insured by benefits plans of large employers.	a) Random design, hospital charts, and records. (b and c) ■ Fee for Service: 1987–present. ■ Encounter: 1994–present. ■ Medicare: 1995–present. ■ Benefit Plan Design (compilation of others): 1993–present.	The cost of obtaining the data sets may be prohibitive.	The Medstat Group. (734) 913-3000 www.medstat.com
Quitline Call Monitoring ■ Provides data on the number of calls to quitlines for counseling and referrals. ■ May provide information on success rates.	*Topics:* ■ Number of calls. ■ Sex and race/ethnicity of callers. ■ Type of cessation information provided.	State level or quitline service area.	a) Varies.		State health departments with quitlines.
Third Party Payer Surveys ■ Tracks insurance coverage and reimbursement.	*Topics:* ■ Coverage for cessation services. ■ Health care provider policies related to tobacco.	National and state payers. *Subjects:* Medicaid, Medicare, private insurers.	a) Varies. b) Not applicable.		Health Care Financing Administration. (800)-Medicare. www.hcfa.gov State health departments.

Table 3 *(continued)*

Abbreviations: COBRA = Consolidated Omnibus Budget Reconciliation Act.

Appendix A

Table 4. Topic-Specific Tools: Sales Data

Data Source	Tobacco-Related Indicators	Sampling Frame	Methodology (a), Frequency (b), Years Completed (c)	Comments	Contact
Food and Drug Administration (FDA) Compliance Checks ■ Provides data on retailers that complied with the prohibition of the sale of tobacco products to minors. ■ Prior to March 21, 2000, the compliance check authorized state and local authorities to survey whether retailers followed the FDA regulation that prohibited the sale of cigarettes and smokeless tobacco to children younger than 18 years.	*Topics:* ■ Ability of minors to purchase tobacco products.	National and state levels. *Subjects:* Local tobacco retailers.	a) Random, unannounced visits by state or local officials authorized by the FDA. Methodology may vary by state. b) Annual. c) 1997–2000.	Supreme Court ruled that FDA exceeded authority. Data collection suspended on March 21, 2000.	Food and Drug Administration. (888) 453-6332. www.fda.gov/opacom/campaigns/tobacco
Scanner Data ■ Provides market data on tobacco sales using universal product code numbers.	*Topics:* ■ Dollar sales. ■ Unit sales. ■ Volume sales. ■ Sales share. ■ Average selling price. ■ Average promoted price. ■ Average list price. ■ Percentage of stores selling each product.	State or local levels. *Subjects:* Retailers using UPC scanners.	a) Varies. c) 1994–present.	Comparable data on grocery stores are available, but the cost of obtaining the data set may be prohibitive.	AC Nielsen and Company. (770) 482-1939. Office on Smoking and Health, Centers for Disease Control and Prevention. (770) 488-5703. www.cdc.gov/tobacco
✓ **Substance Abuse and Mental Health Services Administration (SAMHSA) Compliance Checks** ■ Provides data on tobacco sales to minors through unannounced, annual inspections (includes location of establishments). ■ This monitoring research was authorized through the Synar Amendment, which mandated the reduction of tobacco sales to minors.	*Topics:* ■ Ability of minors to purchase tobacco products.	State and local levels. *Subjects:* Tobacco retailers.	a) Random design. Unannounced visits. Methodology may vary by state. c) 1995–present.	Annual report details states' activities to enforce laws. Includes information on successes in reducing tobacco availability to young people, methods used to identify noncompliant retail outlets, inspection procedures, and plans for enforcing the law in the next fiscal year. Comparability of data may be affected by the race and sex of young inspectors.	Substance Abuse and Mental Health Services Administration. (301) 443-8956. www.samhsa.gov/csap

Table 4
✓Data are frequently used and comparable across states.
Abbreviations: FDA = Food and Drug Administration. UPC = Universal Product Code.

Table 4. Topic-Specific Tools: Sales Data

Data Source	Tobacco-Related Indicators	Sampling Frame	Methodology (a), Frequency (b), Years Completed (c)	Comments	Contact
Tax Revenue Data ■ Provides sales information on tobacco products.	*Topics:* ■ Sales (number of cigarette packs, cartons, and pounds of tobacco) per capita for cigarettes and smokeless tobacco.	State level. *Subjects:* Wholesalers and distributors.	a) Receipts collected monthly. b) Varies by state. Usually begins the first year a state collects tobacco excise tax.	The Tobacco Institute was dismantled in 1999, but Orzechowski and Walker, an economic consulting firm financially supported by tobacco companies, has begun publishing an annual report on tobacco sales and consumption.	Orzechowski and Walker. (703) 351-5014. State departments of revenue.
Tobacco License Database ■ Provides data on establishments approved to sell tobacco products. ■ Can be used for monitoring and enforcement. ■ Provides a sample frame for compliance checks or population observation studies.	*Topics:* ■ Tobacco license or sales permit. ■ Retailer type.	State level. *Subjects:* Tobacco retailers.	a) Varies. b) Varies.		State enforcement or business regulations agency.

Table 4 (continued)

Appendix A

Table 5. Topic-Specific Tools: National, State, and Local Policy Tracking

Data Source	Tobacco-Related Indicators	Sampling Frame	Methodology (a), Frequency (b), Years Completed (c)	Comments	Contact
Restaurant Surveys ■ Provides data on smoking policies and practices; and on the knowledge, behaviors, and attitudes of personnel and/or management.	*Topics:* ■ Type of restaurant. ■ Smoking policy. ■ Reasons for smoking policy. ■ Projected changes in smoking policy. ■ Presence of bar or lounge. ■ Configuration of seating areas. ■ Number of seats in restaurant. ■ Customer demand for smoking or nonsmoking sections. ■ Attitudes about harmfulness of ETS. ■ Support for local smoke-free ordinances. ■ Tobacco use.	State and local levels.	a) Random design using business lists. Methodology may vary by state. c) Most of these surveys have been conducted in the last 10 years.	A limited number of states have conducted this type of survey.	Office on Smoking and Health, Centers for Disease Control and Prevention. (770) 488-5703. www.cdc.gov/tobacco
Worksite Surveys ■ Provides data on prevalence, knowledge, behaviors, attitudes, policies, cessation activities, and practices at private and public work sites.	*Topics:* ■ Tobacco use. ■ Smoking policies in work areas. ■ Smoking policies in common/public places. ■ Attitudes about smoking indoors. ■ Perceptions of the harmfulness of ETS. ■ Cessation policies. ■ Cessation programs.	State and local levels.	a) Random design using business lists. Methodology may vary by state. b) Frequency varies by state.	A limited number of states have conducted this type of survey.	Office on Smoking and Health, Centers for Disease Control and Prevention. (770) 488-5703. www.cdc.gov/tobacco

Table 5

Abbreviations: ETS = environmental tobacco smoke.

Table 7. Topic-Specific Tools: Advertising Tracking and Outcomes Measurement

Data Source	Tobacco-Related Indicators	Sampling Frame	Methodology (a), Frequency (b), Years Completed (c)	Comments	Contact
Arbitron ■ Provides data on which radio stations have the largest reach for the target population. ■ Can be used to target media campaign activities and estimate reach.	*Topics:* ■ Time of day. ■ Amount of time listened. ■ Specific geographical locations. ■ Listener demographics.	Based on county level metropolitan markets.	a) Random design. Mail diary. b) Ongoing, since 1950s.	The biggest metropolitan markets are surveyed four times a year. Smaller markets are surveyed twice a year.	Arbitron. (770) 551-1400 or (800) 543-7300. www.arbitron.com
Media Campaign Activity Tracking ■ Provides tracking data on counter-marketing advertisements on TV and radio.	*Topics:* ■ Gross rating point (GRP) reach and frequency.	Media campaigns.	a) Varies. b) Varies.	This information is usually provided by the media campaign provider or contractor.	State health departments.
Media Evaluation Survey ■ Provides data on the exposure, awareness, and impact of a paid media campaign.	*Topics:* ■ Confirmation of exposure. ■ Recall of specific advertisements. ■ Behavior change.	Target population of media campaign.	a) Random design. Repeated follow-up telephone surveys. b) Varies.	Provides pre- and post-information before, during, and after a counter-marketing campaign. A number of states have mounted counter-marketing campaigns.	Office on Smoking and Health, Centers for Disease Control and Prevention. (770) 488-5703. www.cdc.gov/tobacco State health departments.
Nielsen Sigma Service ■ Provides 24 hours per day tracking of paid and unpaid public service announcements and video news releases. ■ Tracking is done by advertisement master code.	*Topics:* ■ Air time and frequency of advertisement.	Market unit level of advertisements.	a) Census of all full-power commercial broadcasting stations. b) Ongoing since 1989.	Available to ordering client, distribution firm, or organization. The costs obtaining the data sets may be prohibitive.	New Media Services. (727) 738-3060. www.nielsenmedia.com
Video Monitoring Service ■ Tracks broadcast coverage of TV, radio, print, and outdoor advertisements.	*Topics:* ■ Tobacco key words.	Advertisements on TV, radio, print, and outdoors.	a) Census of full-power commercial broadcasting stations. b) Ongoing since 1996.	Number of media sources depends on region.	Video Monitoring Services. (212) 736-2010. www.vidmon.com

Table 7

Table 8. Topic-Specific Tools: Community

Data Source	Tobacco-Related Indicators	Sampling Frame	Methodology (a), Frequency (b), Years Completed (c)	Comments	Contact
Key Informant Surveys ■ Provides data on awareness and attitudes of leaders and influential persons on tobacco issues from various sectors of the community, including law enforcement, business, faith, education, etc.	*Topics:* ■ Importance of tobacco-related issues. ■ Investment in health.	Community level. *Subjects:* Leaders, potential partners, and other influential persons.	a) Varies (e.g., snowball, quota sample, in-person, or telephone survey). b) Varies.	A limited number of states have conducted this type of survey.	State health departments.
Local Program Monitoring ■ Provides data on local tobacco control program infrastructure, staff, resources, and objectives.	*Topics:* ■ Staffing. ■ Resources. ■ Activities.	Local level. *Subjects:* Program manager and project coordinators.	a) Varies (e.g., self-administered progress report) b) Varies.	A limited number of states have conducted this type of survey.	Office on Smoking and Health, Centers for Disease Control and Prevention. (770) 488-5703. www.cdc.gov/tobacco State health departments.

Table 8

Appendix B

Preventing the Initiation of Tobacco Use Among Young People

- Example of Logic Model
- Examples of Outcome and Process Objectives
- Example Outcomes, Outputs, Indicators, and Data Sources

Appendix B

Preventing the Initiation of Tobacco Use Among Young People

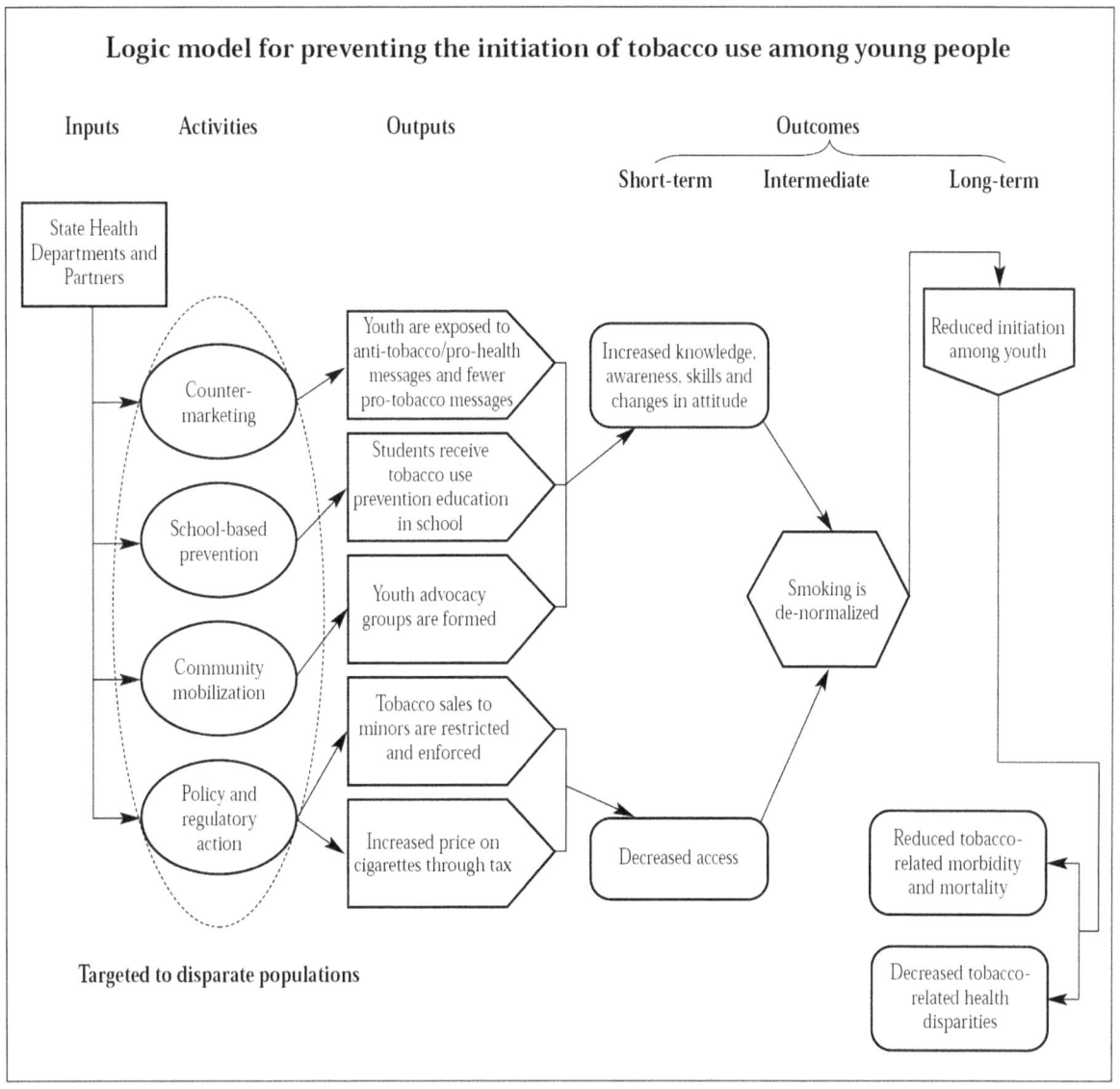

Program goal: prevent tobacco initiation among young people

Examples of outcome objectives

Examples of long-term objectives

- Reduce the proportion of young people in grades 9 through 12 who have used any tobacco product in the previous month from X% in 2001 to Y% in 2005.

- Increase by at least 1 year the average age of first use of cigarettes by adolescents aged 12–17 by 2005.

- Increase the proportion of young people in grades 9 through 12 who report having never tried a cigarette from X% in 2001 to Y% in 2005.

Examples of intermediate objectives

Strategy: Decrease the social acceptability of tobacco use.

- Decrease the proportion of young people who believe that people who smoke have more friends from X% in 2001 to Y% in 2003.

- Decrease the proportion of young people in grades 6 through 8 who definitely feel that smoking cigarettes makes young people look cool or fit in from X% in 2001 to Y% in 2003.

- Decrease the proportion of young people in grades 9 through 12 who definitely feel that smoking cigarettes makes young people look cool or fit in from X% in 2001 to Y% in 2003.

- Decrease the proportion of young people in grades 6 through 8 who would ever use or wear something that has a tobacco company name or picture on it from X% in 2001 to Y% in 2003.

- Decrease the proportion of young people in grades 9 through 12 who would ever use or wear something that has a tobacco company name or picture on it from X% in 2001 to Y% in 2003.

- Increase the number of communities with local ordinances restricting tobacco advertising within 1,000 feet of schools, parks, and playgrounds from X in 2001 to Y in 2003.

Strategy: Decrease young people's access to tobacco.

- Increase the proportion of retailers who refuse to sell to minors from X% in 2001 to Y% in 2003.

- Increase the proportion of young people in grades 9 through 12 who were refused sales of cigarettes during the prior 30 days from X% in 2001 to Y% in 2003.

Examples of short-term objectives

Strategy: Increase young people's awareness and knowledge about the risks of tobacco use; improve their attitudes toward nonsmoking and their skills in resisting tobacco use.

- Increase the proportion of young people in grades 6 through 8 who have seen messages on television, radio, billboards, or other media about not smoking from X% in 2001 to Y% in 2002.

- Increase the proportion of targeted young people in grades 6 through 8 who have seen messages on television, radio, billboards, or other media about not smoking from X% in 2001 to Y% in 2002.

- Increase the proportion of young people in grades 6 through 8 who believe people can get addicted to tobacco from X% in 2001 to Y% in 2002.

- Increase the proportion of young people in grades 6 through 8 who have practiced ways to say "no" to tobacco during the previous school year from X% in 2001 to Y% in 2002.

- Increase the proportion of targeted young people in grades 6 through 8 who have practiced ways to say "no" to tobacco during the past school year from X% in 2001 to Y% in 2002.

- Increase the proportion of young people in grades 9 through 12 who have seen messages on television, radio, billboards, or other media about not smoking from X% in 2001 to Y% in 2002.

- Increase the proportion of young people in grades 9 through 12 who believe people can get addicted to tobacco from X% in 2001 to Y% in 2002.

- Increase the proportion of young people in grades 9 through 12 who have practiced ways to say "no" to tobacco during the previous school year from X% in 2001 to Y% in 2002.

- Increase the proportion of young people in various population groups in grades 9 through 12 who have practiced ways to say "no" to tobacco during the previous school year from X% in 2001 to Y% in 2002.

Strategy: Restrict tobacco sales to minors and enforce laws related to restricting such sales.

- Increase the proportion of smokers in grades 9 through 12 who were asked to show proof of age the last time they attempted to purchase cigarettes from X% in 2001 to Y% in 2002.

- Increase the proportion of smokers in grades 9 through 12 who have ever had a retailer refuse to sell them cigarettes from X% in 2001 to Y% in 2002.

Examples of process objectives

Strategy: Promote school programs to prevent tobacco use.

- By December 2002, conduct teacher training on a tobacco-use-prevention curriculum that is consistent with the CDC recommended guidelines in at least 25% of school districts.

- By September 2003, increase the percentage of school districts that are implementing a tobacco-use-prevention curriculum that meets the CDC recommended guidelines to at least 15%.

Strategy: Promote youth advocacy to empower young people to live a smoke-free lifestyle.

- By June 2002, fund at least five community organizations that primarily serve particular populations of people (e.g, African Americans, blue-collar workers) to develop youth advocacy groups to promote nonsmoking norms.

Strategy: Decrease young people's access to tobacco products.

- By December 2002, conduct tobacco retail compliance checks in at least 10 municipalities in collaboration with youth advocacy groups and police departments.

Appendix B

Example Outcomes, Outputs, Indicators, and Data Sources for the Program Goal of Reducing Tobacco Initiation Among Young People.

Long-Term Outcomes	Long-Term Indicators	Data Sources*
Decreased prevalence of tobacco use among young people.	■ Proportion of young people who report smoking a cigarette in the prior 30 days.	■ Youth Tobacco Survey. ■ Youth Risk Behavior Survey.
Delayed average age at first use.	■ Average age at which young people smoke a whole cigarette for the first time.	■ Youth Tobacco Survey.
Increased prevalence of young people who have never tried a cigarette.	■ Proportion of young people who report they have never tried a cigarette.	■ Youth Tobacco Survey.
Intermediate Outcomes	**Intermediate Indicators**	**Data Sources***
Decreased social acceptance of tobacco use.	■ Proportion of young people who believe smoking does not make them look cool or fit in. ■ Proportion of young people who report they would not wear something that has a tobacco company name or picture on it. ■ Proportion of young people who do not think people who smoke cigarettes have more friends. ■ Number of communities with ordinances restricting tobacco advertising near schools, parks, and playgrounds.	■ Youth Tobacco Survey. ■ DASH School Profile. ■ Copies of ordinances.
Decreased access to tobacco for young people.	■ Proportion of retailers who refuse to sell cigarettes to minors. ■ Proportion of young people who report buying a pack of cigarettes within the prior 30 days.	■ Retailer Survey. ■ Youth Tobacco Survey.
Improved attitudes about smoking among young people.	■ Proportion of young people who report they would not wear or use something with a tobacco name or picture on it. ■ Proportion of young people who believe they can resist peer pressure to smoke. ■ Proportion of young people with a firm intention to never smoke.	■ Youth Tobacco Survey.
Short-Term Outcomes	**Short-Term Indicators**	**Data Sources***
Increased knowledge and awareness about the dangers of smoking.	■ Proportion of young people who believe people can get addicted to tobacco. ■ Proportion of people who recall content of anti-smoking, youth-focused counter-advertisements, brochures, posters, or presentations. ■ Proportion of young people who remember seeing counter-advertisements, brochures, posters, or presentations.	■ Youth Tobacco Survey. ■ State Survey.
Increased skills to reduce tobacco use.	■ Proportion of young people who have been taught during the previous school year to practice ways to say "no" to tobacco.	■ Youth Tobacco Survey.
Increased adoption and enforcement of tobacco-free school policies.	■ Proportion of schools that have implemented school-based tobacco prevention programs. ■ Proportion of young people who report smoking on school property within the prior 30 days.	■ DASH School Profile. ■ Youth Tobacco Survey.
Increased restriction and enforcement of tobacco sales to minors.	■ Proportion of young people who report retailers refused to sell cigarettes to them. ■ Proportion of young people who report being asked for proof of age by retailers when purchasing cigarettes.	■ Youth Tobacco Survey.

Abbreviations: DASH = CDC's Division of Adolescent and School Health.

Example Outcomes, Outputs, Indicators, and Data Sources for the Program Goal of Reducing Tobacco Initiation Among Young People

Process Outcomes	Process Indicators	Data Sources*
Increased number of schools with programs to prevent tobacco use.	■ Percentage of school districts that have conducted teacher training on a CDC-recommended tobacco-use-prevention curriculum. ■ Percentage of school districts that have implemented a CDC-recommended tobacco-use-prevention curriculum.	■ Site-specific survey of school districts. ■ DASH School Profile
Increased number of youth advocacy groups whose purpose is to empower young people to say "*no*" to tobacco.	■ Number of contracts with ethnic-minority community organizations to develop youth advocacy groups for the purpose of helping young people not to smoke.	■ Copies of contracts. ■ NTCP-Chronicle Progress Report.
Decreased access of young people to tobacco products.	■ Number of communities in which tobacco retail compliance checks were completed.	■ State or local progress reports.

Abbreviations: DASH = CDC's Division of Adolescent and School Health; NTCP = CDC's National Tobacco Control Program

Appendix C

Promoting Smoking Cessation Among Young People and Adults

- Example of Logic Model
- Examples of Outcome and Process Objectives
- Example Outcomes, Outputs, Indicators, and Data Sources

Appendix C

Promoting Smoking Cessation Among Young People and Adults

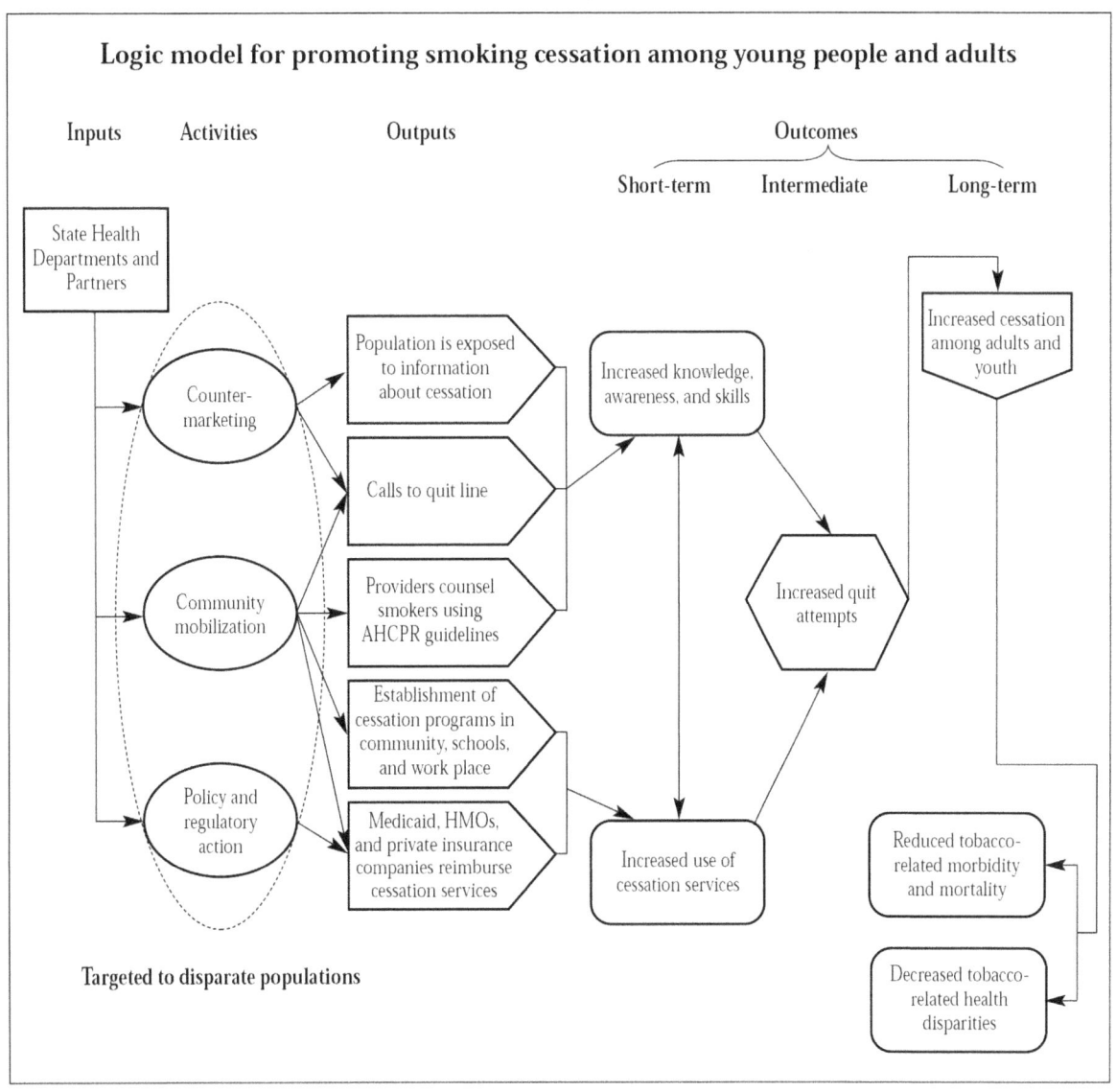

Program goal: promote smoking cessation among young people and adults

Examples of outcome objectives

Examples of long-term objectives

- In state X, increase the proportion of adults who report they have quit smoking in the prior 12 months from X% in 2001 to Y% in 2005.

- In state X, increase the proportion of adolescent smokers who report they did not smoke cigarettes in the prior 6 months from X% in 2001 to Y% in 2005.

Strategy: Decrease smoking rate among pregnant women.

- Increase the proportion of women smokers who did not smoke in the last 3 months of pregnancy and remained abstinent through postpartum from X% in 2001 to Y% in 2005.

- Increase the proportion of target-population women smokers who did not smoke in the last 3 months of pregnancy and remained abstinent through postpartum from X% in 2001 to Y% in 2005.

Examples of intermediate objectives

Strategy: Increase the rate of quit attempts.

- Increase the proportion of adult smokers who, in the previous year, made at least one quit attempt that lasted longer than 24 hours from X% in 2001 to Y% in 2003.

- Increase the proportion of smokers in grades 9 through 12 who have tried to quit smoking in the previous 12 months from X% to Y% in 2003.

- Increase the proportion of target-population smokers in grades 9 through 12 who have tried to quit smoking in the previous 12 months from X% to Y% in 2003.

Strategy: Increase the percentage of smokers who intend to quit.

- Increase the percentage of adult smokers who report they would like to quit smoking from X% in 2001 to Y% in 2003.

- Increase the percentage of adult smokers who report they are seriously considering quitting smoking within the next 6 months from X% in 2002 to Y% in 2003.

Appendix C

- Increase the percentage of target-population adult smokers who report they are seriously considering quitting smoking within the next 6 months from X% in 2002 to Y% in 2003.

- Increase the percentage of young people in grades 9 through 12 who report they are seriously considering quitting smoking within the next 6 months from X% in 2002 to Y % in 2003.

- Increase the percentage of target-population young people in grades 9 through 12 who report they are seriously considering quitting smoking within the next 6 months from X% in 2002 to Y% in 2003.

Strategy: Promote smoking-cessation programs in workplaces and other community settings.

- Increase the proportion of smokers who report their workplace offers formal smoking-cessation programs from X% in 2001 to Y % in 2002.

- Increase the proportion of smokers in particular groups (e.g., Hispanics, pregnant women) who report their workplace offers formal smoking-cessation programs from X% in 2001 to Y% in 2002.

- Increase the percentage of minority-owned businesses offering formal workplace smoking-cessation programs from X% in 2001 to Y% in 2002.

- Increase the proportion of smokers who can identify at least one smoking-cessation resource from which they could receive help from X% in 2001 to Y% in 2002.

- Increase the proportion of smokers who know about a quitline from X% in 2001 to Y% in 2002.

Strategy: Encourage health care providers to counsel patients to quit using tobacco.

- Increase the proportion of health care providers who routinely counsel their tobacco-using patients to quit from X% in 2001 to Y% in 2002.

- Increase the proportion of adult smokers who report that a doctor or other health care professional advised them to quit smoking during the previous 12 months from X% in 2001 to Y% in 2002.

Strategy: Increase the proportion of health insurance plans that offer cessation services.

- Increase the proportion of health insurance plans that offer smoking-cessation services as a covered benefit from X% in 2001 to Y% in 2002.

- Increase the proportion of health insurance plans that offer pharmaceutical treatment of nicotine addiction as a covered benefit from X% in 2001 to Y% in 2002.

Examples of short-term objectives

Strategy: Improve awareness, knowledge, and attitudes related to cessation among adult smokers.

- Increase the proportion of adult smokers who recall the content of cessation advertising, brochures, posters, or presentations from X% in 2001 to Y% in 2002.

- Increase the proportion of a particular group of adult smokers (e.g., Hispanics, low-literacy groups, gays and lesbians) who recall the content of cessation advertising, brochures, posters, or presentations from X% in 2001 to Y% in 2002.

- Increase the proportion of adult smokers who believe quitting smoking is beneficial to their health from X% in 2001 to Y% in 2002.

- Increase the proportion of adult smokers who are confident they would be able to quit smoking permanently from X% in 2001 to Y% in 2002.

Strategy: Improve awareness, knowledge, and attitudes related to cessation among health care system staff, health care professionals, and insurance purchasers (e.g., businesses, managed care organizations, business coalitions, Medicaid staff, state employee benefits managers).

- Increase the proportion of health care system staff that receive training on reminder systems from X% in 2001 to Y% in 2002.

- Increase the proportion of insurers and purchasers of insurance who receive briefings on insurance coverage from X% in 2001 to Y% in 2002.

- Increase the proportion of insurers and purchasers of insurance who receive model descriptions of insurance benefits from X% in 2001 to Y% in 2002.

Examples of process objectives

Strategy: Promote smoking-cessation programs.

- By October 2001, have at least three local coalitions with Web sites that list smoking-cessation programs in their communities.

- By June 2002, establish new smoking-cessation programs in at least five rural communities with no prior cessation resources.

Strategy: Promote health systems change

- By February 2002, meet with decision makers from at least two managed care plans to provide the rationale for covering smoking-cessation benefits through their employer-funded plans.

- By May 2002, distribute chart stickers for tracking patient tobacco use through at least five county medical societies.

Strategy: Promote decreased social acceptability of tobacco use.

- By August 2002, develop a media campaign, with materials tailored to the target population, that encourages adults and adolescents to quit smoking to improve their health.

Example Outcomes, Outputs, Indicators, and Data Sources for the Program Goal of Increasing Smoking Cessation Among Young People and Adults

Long-Term Outcomes	Long-Term Indicators	Data Sources*
Increased nonsmoking during pregnancy.	■ Proportion of women who report smoking less than one cigarette a day during the prior 3 months of their pregnancy. ■ Proportion of women who report smoking 3 months before pregnancy and not smoking after pregnancy.	■ Pregnancy Risk Assessment Monitoring System.
Increased smoking cessation.	■ Percentage of adult smokers who report quitting in the prior year. ■ Percentage of young smokers who report quitting in past 6 months.	■ Behavioral Risk Factor Surveillance System, optional module. ■ Youth Tobacco Survey.
Intermediate Outcomes	**Intermediate Indicators**	**Data Sources***
Increased quit attempts.	■ Percentage of adult smokers who stopped smoking for 1 day or longer in the prior 12 months in an attempt to quit smoking. ■ Percentage of adolescent smokers who tried to quit smoking cigarettes during the prior 12 months.	■ Behavioral Risk Factor Surveillance System, optional module. ■ Youth Tobacco Survey. ■ Adult Tobacco Survey.
Increased intentions to quit.	■ Percentage of adult smokers who report they would like to quit smoking. ■ Percentage of adult smokers who report they are seriously considering quitting within the next 6 months. ■ Percentage of adolescent smokers who report they would like to quit smoking.	■ Adult Tobacco Survey. ■ Youth Tobacco Survey.
Short-Term Outcomes	**Short-Term Indicators**	**Data Sources***
Improved awareness, knowledge, attitude, and skills related to smoking cessation.	■ Proportion of adults who recall the content of cessation PSAs, brochures, posters, or presentations. ■ Proportion of adult smokers who believe quitting smoking is beneficial to their health. ■ Proportion of adults who are confident they could quit smoking permanently.	■ Adult Tobacco Survey. ■ State-specific surveys.
Increased availability of cessation programs in wide variety of settings.	■ Proportion of adolescent smokers who report participation in a program to help them quit using tobacco. ■ Proportion of pregnant women who report attending classes on how to stop smoking. ■ Proportion of smokers who report their workplace offers a smoking-cessation program. ■ Proportion of adults who can identify at least one smoking-cessation resource from which they could receive help.	■ Youth Tobacco Survey. ■ Pregnancy Risk Assessment Monitoring System. ■ Adult Tobacco Survey.
Increased smoking-cessation counseling by health care providers.	■ Proportion of adult smokers who have been advised to quit smoking by a health care professional in the prior 12 months. ■ Proportion of women who report a health care professional spoke to them during prenatal visits about how smoking can harm their baby.	■ BRFSS optional module. ■ Pregnancy Risk Assessment Monitoring System. ■ Adult Tobacco Survey.
Increased coverage of cessation services in health insurance plans.	■ Proportion of health insurance plans that cover smoking-cessation services. ■ Proportion of health insurance plans that cover treatment of nicotine addiction.	■ State surveys.

Appendix C

Example Outcomes, Outputs, Indicators, and Data Sources for Programs with a Goal of Increasing Smoking Cessation Among Young People and Adults

Process Outcomes	Process Indicators	Data Sources*
Increased availability of smoking-cessation programs.	■ Number of Web sites listing community smoking-cessation services. ■ Number of new smoking-cessation programs offered in rural communities.	■ State or local progress reports.
Increased greater attention to smoking-cessation by health care systems.	■ Number of meetings with managed care plans about adding coverage of smoking-cessation. ■ Number of county medical societies distributing chart stickers for tracking patient tobacco use.	■ State or local progress reports. ■ Copies of meeting agendas.
Decreased acceptability of tobacco use.	■ Copies of media spots developed as part of the media campaign to promote smoking cessation.	■ State or local progress reports.

Appendix D

Evaluation Contracts Checklist

Evaluation Contracts Checklist

Daniel L. Stufflebeam, February 2001

Instructions: Mark each item as *important and incorporated* with a checkmark or *not applicable (na)* or leave it blank, indicating *not agreed to though important*.

1. Basic Considerations
- _____ Object of the evaluation
- _____ Purpose of the evaluation
- _____ Client
- _____ Other right-to-know audiences
- _____ Authorized evaluator(s)
- _____ Guiding values and criteria
- _____ Standards for judging the evaluation
- _____ Contractual questions

2. Information
- _____ Required information
- _____ Data-collection procedures
- _____ Data-collection instruments and protocols
- _____ Information sources
- _____ Participant selection
- _____ Provisions to obtain needed permissions to collect data
- _____ Follow-up procedures to assure adequate information
- _____ Provisions for assuring the quality of obtained information
- _____ Provisions to store and maintain security of collected information

3. Analysis
- _____ Procedures for analyzing quantitative information
- _____ Procedures for analyzing qualitative information

4. Synthesis
- _____ Participants in the process to reach judgments
- _____ Procedures and guidelines for synthesizing findings and reaching judgments
- _____ Decisions on whether evaluation reports should include recommendations

5. Reports
- _____ Deliverables and due dates
- _____ Interim report formats, contents, lengths, audiences, and methods of delivery
- _____ Final report format, contents, length, audiences, and methods of delivery
- _____ Restrictions/permissions to publish information from or based on the evaluation

---

> **Working with contractors**
>
> This checklist will help program managers, staff, evaluators, and evaluation clients identify key contractual issues and make and record their agreements for conducting an evaluation. Advance agreements on these matters can mean the difference between an evaluation's success and failure.

6. Reporting Safeguards
_____ Anonymity/confidentiality
_____ Prerelease review of reports
_____ Conditions for participating in prerelease reviews
_____ Rebuttal by evaluatees
_____ Editorial authority
_____ Final authority to release reports

7. Protocol
_____ Contact persons
_____ Rules for contacting program personnel
_____ Communication channels and assistance

8. Evaluation Management
_____ Time line for evaluation work of both clients and evaluators
_____ Assignment of evaluation responsibilities

9. Client Responsibilities
_____ Access to information
_____ Services
_____ Personnel
_____ Information
_____ Facilities
_____ Equipment
_____ Materials
_____ Transportation assistance
_____ Workspace

10. Evaluation Budget
_____ Payment amounts and dates
_____ Conditions for payment, including delivery of required reports
_____ Budget limits/restrictions
_____ Agreed-upon indirect/overhead rates
_____ Contracts for budgetary matters

11. Review and Control of the Evaluation
_____ Contract amendment and cancellation provisions
_____ Provisions for periodic review, modification, and renegotiation of the evaluation design as needed
_____ Provision for evaluating the evaluation against professional standards of sound evaluation

---

Reprinted with permission from:
The Evaluation Center
Western Michigan University
Kalamazoo, MI 49008-5237
Eval-Center@wmich.edu
www.wmich.edu/evalctr/index.html

www.ingramcontent.com/pod-product-compliance
Lightning Source LLC
Chambersburg PA
CBHW081726170526
45167CB00009B/3722